Praise for Ali Katz

"Ali writes with candor, clarity, and courage. . . . You know you have a friend who walks this journey to self-love with you."

—Sarah McLean, author of *Soul-Centered: Transform Your Life in 8 Weeks with Meditation*

"With honest, compassionate stories, Katz provides parents with life-affirming tools; a road map to come back to their core essence and highest parenting purpose."

—Michele Kambolis, registered clinical counselor and author of *Generation Stressed*

"Everyone has different ways of living a healthy life, but Ali Katz has it down to a science . . . [she] leaves you with a feeling of hope and a feeling that *if Ali can do it, so can I*, because you see that she practices what she preaches."

—*Just Vibe*

"We get to experience her journey and learn, as she did, how to grow deeper in ourselves and become a little bit better each and every day in order to enjoy the simple times with our children and spread our happiness to them."

—*Modern Mom*

"Ali is a breath of fresh air amidst the crazy world of parenting and family life. These bite-sized lessons are so transformative; I saw results in my life!"

—Robyn Youkilis, author of *Go With Your Gut* and founder of *Your Healthiest You* blog

"Ali gave us so many wonderful takeaways on how to begin your own meditation practice and how to create mindfulness with meditation. We know you are going to love it!"

—*Strong Body Whole Heart* podcast

One Minute
to
Zen

Go From Hot Mess to Mindful Mom
in One Minute or Less

Ali Katz

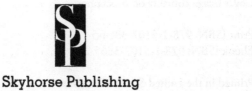

Skyhorse Publishing

Skyhorse Publishing books may be purchased in bulk at special discounts for sales promotion, corporate gifts, fund-raising, or educational purposes. Special editions can also be created to specifications. For details, contact the Special Sales Department, Skyhorse Publishing, 307 West 36th Street, 11th Floor, New York, NY 10018 or info@skyhorsepublishing.com.

Skyhorse® and Skyhorse Publishing® are registered trademarks of Skyhorse Publishing, Inc.®, a Delaware corporation.

Visit our website at www.skyhorsepublishing.com.

10 9 8 7 6 5 4 3 2 1

Library of Congress Cataloging-in-Publication Data is available on file.

Cover design by Mona Lin
Cover image courtesy of iStockphoto

Print ISBN: 978-1-5107-3864-5
Ebook ISBN: 978-1-5107-3865-2

Printed in the United States of America

Contents

Introduction

There are no coincidences in life, only synchronicities, and I believe that with my whole being. Situations keep happening in my life that only strengthen this comforting way of thinking, and here is a perfect example.

The week I signed the contract with my publisher to write this book I was diagnosed with inflammatory arthritis. Truth be told, I did have warning—even if I didn't see it at the time, which has turned into a very cool story that I'm excited to share. I now feel more secure owning my truth and connection to spirit, which is not what this book is about, but it's part of who I am, and I like to put it all out there. If you read my first two books, you already know this about me!

Two weeks before my diagnosis I was lying in bed savoring the delicious, albeit brief moment between asleep and awake. I heard a voice as clear as a bell in my head that said, "You have rheumatoid arthritis, and you need to see a doctor. Go see Holly Wade."

So much made sense in that moment, and I realized that all the weird symptoms I had been feeling over the past few months were not in my head. I was obviously not clueing in at all, and I think my angels were like, "She doesn't get it! We need to make this *really* clear." I'll never forget that voice in my head, softening the blow of the word "arthritis." I was so excited about hearing such a crystal-clear clairaudient message that the arthritis bit wasn't what I was focusing on in that first moment. I was just celebrating the fact that I got the message in general, as ridiculous as that may sound now!

I immediately understood why my hands were so stiff every morning, and the excuse I made that I kept banging the knuckle on my middle finger was ridiculous. I'm not sure how I even could have, but that's what I kept telling myself when it was terribly sore. Some of my knuckles would be so sore holding on to my dogs' leashes that I'd have to cut walks short. I remember a week before I heard this message from my angel I told my husband, "It hurts so much to walk the dogs, you'd think I have arthritis or something!" Ummm . . . think my intuition was kicking in there?

When I hopped out of bed that morning my first thought was, *Of course! It must be rheumatoid arthritis. Why didn't I think of that!* and then I ran downstairs to the drawer in my office where I keep business cards.

Six years ago, I had to see a rheumatologist about a different matter and I went to find her card. Her name is Dr. Holly Jones, not Holly Wade, but the Holly was there and that was confirmation enough for me. I made an appointment that morning for her first available two weeks later.

During those two weeks of waiting I thanked my angels profusely and greedily asked for more messages just like that, so loud and clear. I also began to adjust to the realization that I had another autoimmune disease in addition to my thyroid condition that I had been managing for thirteen years.

I only let myself go onto Google once and only for a minute. I had all of the major symptoms, including exhaustion. I was so tired some days I thought I was going to pass out—at least now I knew why!

Every time I started to worry about my symptoms I took a moment to breathe. Every time I worried about what the doctor would say I remembered to breathe. I was doing one-minute meditations all day long to keep myself in the present moment. Worrying wasn't going to change anything, it would only steal the joy from my present, so what was the point? Everyone's body is different and my plan was to stay as healthy as possible for as long as possible.

For years I have been incorporating one-minute meditations into my day, but I needed them in a whole new way with this revelation. That's when it hit me. It turned out I was writing this book as much for me as for you.

One-minute meditations have been my saving grace through my kids fighting, daily mom overwhelm, frustration, anger, sadness, worry, people annoying me, and managing life in general. They were also my savior through a medical diagnosis.

I am thrilled to be sharing the tools that help me to manage my day-to-day life and live with more ease. These tools are meant to be used throughout your day in times of stress, but also in times where you simply want to create a mindful moment for yourself or a little zen.

I hope you love them and use them as much as I do.

SECTION 1

Perspective Is Key

The Beginning of Everything

If you change the way you look at things, the things you look at change."
—DR. WAYNE DYER

Life demands more from us every day, from the political climate and natural disasters to cranky kids. Moms need ways to deal with stress swiftly and with ease. I hope this book becomes your trusty "calm mom guidebook" of sorts. I have filled it with easy-to-remember and simple-to-practice tools, which are just what you need when dealing with, well, life in general.

Life feels overwhelming and exhausting much of the time, which is why these thirty-five tools are designed to help deal with stress in one minute (the same amount of time it can take for all hell to break loose!).

So many people tell me, "I can't sit still," or "I can't meditate." I can assure you that you can do *anything* for one minute! Meditation feels so hard because most people put unrealistic expectations on themselves when it comes to what a meditation is actually supposed to be or feel like.

Before we jump in, we need to cover some important groundwork that can shift your perspective in many ways. Perspective is everything, so as tempting as it is to skip ahead, don't sell yourself short! Honor yourself and decide which of these changes and shifts will benefit you. Gaining more awareness around these issues is paramount to real change. You can do it!

Meditation can help you regain mental clarity and make you feel more equipped to deal with life's up and downs and even the many demands of your everyday life. It creates feelings of inner peace and wellbeing, helps with decision making, and increases compassion for ourselves and others. You can boost your immune system, heighten your creativity, and lower your risk of disease. Is meditation sounding better to you yet?

There are numerous scientific studies on the effects of meditation. You can pretty much Google anything and "meditation" and it will tell you how it helps. A study was done at Harvard that showed that a short daily meditation increased the gray matter in our brains in areas impacting self-awareness. It decreased gray matter in the brain in areas associated with negative stress.

A study done at Yale University showed the brains of people who meditated consistently develop a new default mode—one of more lasting, present, centered awareness. Imagine if when a stressful situation happened, your first instinct was to take a deep breath and stay calm!

Most scientific studies are based on ten to twenty minutes of meditation using it as a preventative tool, sort of like taking a daily vitamin. Meditation can also be used prescriptively, like taking a Tylenol if you have a headache. That's what all of the one-minute meditations I am going to share with you will do. A mindful pause can halt the stress response and activate your rest-and-digest response, which means your body is operating optimally. I will dive more into stress and what it does to your body in Chapter 2.

One-minute meditations can be done anywhere at any time. You can have your eyes open or closed depending on your situation, and nobody around you even has to know what you are doing! These are the most portable self-help and self-care tools in the world. Once you start using them you won't be able to imagine your life without them and you will be managing stress one mindful minute at a time.

Each new breath we take is another opportunity to decide how the next moment will unfold. If we don't like how we felt a second ago, we have the ability to change directions immediately. Our breath happens in the present moment, so using it in various ways is the ideal way to come back to center.

When my ten-year-old son heard I was writing my third book he asked me, "You still have more to say?!" I chuckled and told him I did, miraculously, have more to say.

As I work with women from across the country, I find that they crave ideas for how to deal with stress in the moment living in this fast-paced world. The most popular speech I give around the country is called "How to Deal with Stress in One Minute or Less," and that's when I knew that no matter what, this book had to be written. I can't keep these tools to myself. They are just too good!

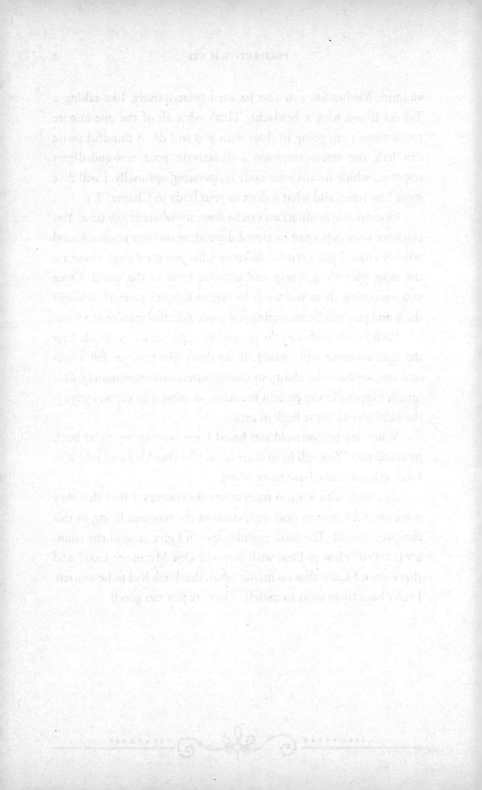

Chapter 1

Your Journey Starts Now

Accepting Where You Are in This Moment

A joyful life is not the result of perfection, but rather of self-compassion."
—JODI BARETZ, THERAPIST AND AUTHOR

The more women I teach, the more I see patterns repeating themselves. It doesn't matter if I'm in a meditation class or in a corporate setting, it's always the same. Women, especially moms, beat themselves up. A lot.

So much time is spent talking and thinking about what they didn't do or what else they need to do. If it's meditation, they aren't consistent enough. If it's healthy eating, they fall off the wagon. If it's spending quality time with their kids, it's spotty. I understand—balancing everything we want to do in a day is *hard*, but judging yourself doesn't help, and it isn't going to change anything. It's just going to make you feel like crap.

Accepting where you are in this moment is the first key to success.

Instead of thinking about all the time you wasted *not* meditating, how about you celebrate the fact that you closed your eyes for a minute and took a mindful pause? All that matters is what you do now. It's never too late to make a change in your life, and I can't think of a better one. Meditation changed my life in the most amazing ways.

I tell all my clients that it's about progress, not perfection. Perfection is an illusion. What's perfect anyway? Who sets that standard?

Small acts lead to big change. The goal is to be a little bit better than you were yesterday, to gain even a miniscule amount more awareness as to what works in your life and what doesn't, and to accept yourself as you are. This doesn't happen in one fell swoop. This happens moment to moment as you make better choices and decisions that feel good in your core. This happens when you use tools to get to know yourself in a whole new way.

When we accept where we are in this moment we can release regret and expectations alike and be present to our life now. We can't change the past, and we can't predict the future, so why do we give them so much power over our happiness?

You are just where you are meant to be in this moment. I really do believe that to be true. Every experience that has come before, both exciting and sad, comfortable and uncomfortable, and everything in between, was necessary to get you *right here.*

When we stop wishing that things were different, the real work can begin. We can bring our energy to what matters instead of ruminating about the past or worrying about the future. We can place our focus on our body, mind, and spirit—on our growth and our loved ones.

Can you commit to yourself in this way? Are you ready for your expansion into living a more mindful life? I promise if you use the tools laid out in this book it is easier to achieve success than you think! If so, make this commitment to yourself and silently repeat:

"I am just where I need to be. I accept myself in this moment. I believe I am worthy of living my very best life which I can do when I commit to myself and make these practices a priority in my life. I am willing and excited. I am ready."

I love this quote by the inspirational author, Anthony D'Angelo: "The greatest gift you can give to yourself is a bit of your own attention." That is what you are about to do, one mindful minute at a time.

When you don't have time, or don't feel like meditating, is often when you need it the most. Another perspective shift can happen around this. We don't find the time for important acts of self-care, we make the time! I dive deep into this in my first two books, but I want to revisit this topic in terms of meditation now.

Meet yourself where you are right here. Can you commit to one minute of meditation at a time? I know you can! By the end of this book you will have tons of options for what to do in one minute to find more calm and peace in your day and how to take the next steps if you want more.

As you make these tools a part of your daily life, and you slowly begin to notice changes in your feelings and behavior, your "why" will emerge. You will be able to finish this sentence in approximately two seconds flat: "I use one-minute meditations because they help me to _____."

When you connect with your "why" it helps you to stay committed and solidify your healthy habits so that they're ingrained into your life to where you practice them automatically. I promise this isn't far off, but the tools only work if you work them. That is so important, let me say it again: *the tools only work if you work them.* So let's get started!

Chapter 2

What Stress Does to Our Bodies

It Can Turn a Regular Moment into a Shit Show

> If stress burned calories, I'd be a supermodel.
>
> —ANONYMOUS

Let's investigate stress a bit, because when we begin to notice how stress feels in our bodies we can become more attuned to how we feel and bring our awareness to refocusing our attention.

The following exercise in stress will give you a better understanding of what stress feels like in your body and what your patterns around stress are.

I'd like you to close your eyes for a moment and think about a stressful situation. It could be an issue in a relationship, a financial responsibility, or anything else. Picture it in your mind's eye and ask yourself the following questions slowly. Give yourself a moment to tune into your body and emotions and let the answers emerge:

- How do you know you are stressed?
- What do you feel in your body?

- How do you treat yourself in this situation?
- How do you treat others?

Now imagine a situation where you are really relaxed. Maybe you are on a beach, or in the mountains, or reading in bed. Ask yourself:

- How does your body feel now?
- How do you treat yourself in this situation?
- How do you treat others?

Those are very different feelings, aren't they?

The very first step in changing how responsive versus reactive we are in moments of stress is acknowledging the sensations in our body, which really clue us in to our emotions. We can become so accustomed to feeling stress that it becomes our sense of normal. We don't really notice we're stressed because we live in a constant state of overwhelm. These feelings don't stand out anymore, and we can't change anything without first being aware of the problem. Ignorance is not bliss when it comes to our emotional state.

What Happens When Stress Builds Up in Your Body?

Andrew Bernstein, the author of *The Myth of Stress,* explains the evolution of stress in really simple terms:

> Once upon a time, as the story goes, our ancestors walked across the grassy plains, only to be confronted by . . . a saber-toothed tiger. These ancestors immediately experienced a hormonal surge, which you may remember from high-school biology as the fight-or-flight response. This response is meant to keep us safe. Faced with a saber-toothed tiger, one had to decide if they were going to fight the tiger or run away.

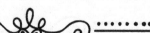

Those who had a strong fight-or-flight response were more likely to survive and produce offspring. Those who didn't have a strong response, for obvious reasons, were not. And so, over the course of many generations, this response was strengthened, eventually becoming hardwired in us as a very useful adaptation. And then something unusual happened.

Life on Earth changed.

Civilizations formed. Villages, then towns, then cities appeared. And, in the space of a few thousand years—the mere blink of an eye from an evolutionary perspective—those grassy plains and saber-toothed tigers were replaced by superhighways and micromanaging bosses. And our fight-or-flight response, calibrated so well to respond to occasional threats, started going haywire.

And that, supposedly, is why we experience so much stress today . . . Our bodies react as if threats are everywhere, as if saber-toothed tigers have us surrounded. We have become victims of our own biology. And the best we can do (we are told) is breathe, relax, exercise, and try to cope.

Our fight-or-flight response kicks in the very same way no matter if someone cuts us off on the freeway, we have a tight work deadline, we see a scary movie, or we imagine something bad happening in our mind. The very same chemical reaction takes place in our body no matter what the stress is.

When stress occurs, chemicals are released in the body:

- Adrenaline sharpens your senses and increases your heart rate and blood pressure, allowing more blood to be sent to your muscles.

- Cortisol acts as an anti-inflammatory.
- Glucagon feeds your muscles more sugar.
- Your breath rate increases to help oxygenate the body.
- Blood is shunted from digestive and sex organs and sent to the heart, lungs, and extremities.
- Your body starts to sweat to keep you cool.
- Platelets get stickier so they can clot better.
- Your immune system refocuses from long-term threats to immediate threats.

That's a lot of chemicals being released and a big-time reaction!

When we feel stress it can take up to four hours for our body to recover and once again be functioning in our preferred rest-and-digest state. So we can be in a state of stress or recovering from it for most of the day. This wreaks havoc on the systems in our body, especially when it happens day in and day out.

According to the Mayo Clinic, the buildup of these hormones in the body from constant stress causes toxicity and can have long term effects, including:

- Heart disease
- Obesity and diabetes
- Allergies
- Reduced immunity
- Infertility
- Digestive troubles
- Headaches
- Insomnia
- Depression
- Anxiety

- Addictions
- Cancer

According to an article in *Psychology Today*, doctors claim that stress is responsible for up to 90 percent of illness and disease. That is an astounding statistic! This number makes you really sit up, take notice, and commit to change.

This is all very shocking, but fortunately I have ways that you can empower yourself to handle the stress in your life better. You don't have to throw your hands up in the air and think there's nothing you can do about it except eventually get sick. You can invest your time and energy into tools that help.

There are ways to create a new normal in our lives, one where our body is in the rest-and-digest mode more than the fight-or-flight response.

What Is Rest and Digest?

When we are in rest and digest, the parasympathetic nervous system, responsible for resting and digestion, is activated and allows the body to operate optimally. Things happen like:

- Secretions of stress hormones decrease
- "Feel-good hormones" such as oxytocin increase
- Heart rate normalizes
- Circulation improves
- The youth hormone DHEA increases
- Digestion and fertility improves

I don't know about you, but I feel more relaxed just reading that list!

There are three optimal ways for your body to deal with stress, and I call them "The Magic Three." They are:

- Sleep
- Exercise
- Meditation

Meditation is usually the one missing for most people, which is where I come in. Enter Ali!

What's amazing about meditation is that it actually changes your brain. I am not going to throw too many scientific terms at you, but it is important to understand that consistent meditation creates neuroplasticity, which means that with consistent practice you can change the way your brain is wired and fires. How cool is that?

Emotional Awareness and Communication

Meditation helps to increase the folds in the insula, the part of your brain that is responsible for emotional connectedness to yourself and others. When this happens, you are better able to listen and communicate effectively and can interpret feedback as a growth opportunity instead of criticism. An experience recently showed me just how true this is.

I had a meeting with someone in the meditation field who I had never met before. We both live in Houston, so it seemed like a nice idea to connect and get to know each other a bit. I'd heard many great things and was really excited to meet her. During our time together, she gave me a big piece of unsolicited advice. I was caught off guard, which made my reaction that much more noticeable.

Pre-meditation, I would say in all honesty that unsolicited advice

would put me majorly on the defensive and cause me to shut down. I can also think of situations where I got defensive and wanted to prove my position or point. This is not a flattering reaction, but many times when it happened I felt defenseless against it. This case was different, though. I was able to remain calm inside and truly listen to what she had to say. Instead of getting defensive and huffy, I ended up feeling really grateful for what she shared. I appreciated her viewpoint, and I felt proud of the growth that I saw in myself. Win/win.

Less Reactive, More Responsive

Meditation helps to decrease gray matter in the amygdala, the part of our brain that controls our fight-or-flight response, which is responsible for fear, anxiety, and stress. When this happens, we become less reactive and more responsive.

We can stop wishing for so many do-overs which translates to less screaming at the kids and then feeling terrible afterward, or wishing you had thought more about that text before you sent it. Not that these situations never happen again, but they are definitely fewer and farther between.

Learning, Focus, and Memory

A consistent meditation practice also helps to increase gray matter in the hippocampus, which is responsible for learning and memory. For this reason, meditation is incredible for people of all ages. Children benefit from meditation, so be sure to teach your kids as many of the one-minute meditations as they want to learn. Share with your own parents that even the Alzheimer's Association advocates for daily meditation, and since we are all going to inevitably age, this study is important for us all to understand.

A study done at UCLA found that a three-month course of yoga and meditation practice helped minimize the cognitive and emotional problems that often precede Alzheimer's disease and other forms of dementia—and that it was even more effective than the memory enhancement exercises that had once been considered the gold standard for managing mild cognitive impairment. How cool is that?

I get so jazzed about meditation because it is the most portable self-care and self-help tool we have. You will read this fact a few times because I really want it to hit home that it is always available to us, and it doesn't cost a dime! It's simple, effective, and can be done anywhere at any time. Meditation works whether you are on a zafu cushion, hiding in a bathroom stall, or taking a few minutes to regroup in your car. And it can be preventive or prescriptive.

Preventive and Prescriptive

Taking a vitamin every day keeps you healthy, just like having a daily seated meditation practice has amazing benefits for the body, mind, and spirit. It keeps you on an even keel, feeling more centered and balanced.

Dr. Sara Lazar, of Harvard University, puts it really simply, "Meditating is like going to the gym. The more you go, the stronger, fitter, and younger your brain."

My personal meditation experience started with eight minutes a day for eight weeks. I noticed the first change in myself after six weeks. I will never forget the moment when I was walking my dog and I stopped short. You see, I lived with anxiety that felt like a brick on my chest for years. I was so used to it, and it was just a part of my existence. I stopped short because all of a sudden I realized in that moment that that brick had lifted, and I finally felt free.

At first I wondered, *Where did it go?* Then I laughed out loud and asked myself, *Who cares?* I realized that the only thing different in my life was that I was meditating, so I decided to keep going and as time went on I noticed more benefits; I felt more compassion toward myself and others, I didn't yell as much, I felt more confident and connected to my intuition, and I was able to sleep better.

Sometimes, even though you adhere to a preventative lifestyle, you can get a headache during the day, and you need a Tylenol. You need something to help in the moment. That would be a prescriptive response to something you feel right now. *That is what a one-minute meditation does for your nervous system. It calms it in the moment of stress and brings you back to center and balance.*

I wake up and meditate every day, but I also use mediation in moments of stress throughout the day, just like I would take a Tylenol if I had a headache.

I don't have four hours to recover from stress on my way to a see a client if someone cuts me off as they cross three lanes of traffic on the freeway and absolutely ignore the fact that I am simply driving in my lane. I need to stop stress in its tracks so that I can arrive wherever I am going with my positive energy intact, and that's just what happens when I use a quick meditation while stopped at a traffic light after I exit the freeway. Houston traffic definitely gives me plenty of time to practice!

If I am having a judgmental thought about myself or someone else I can stop it cold in just a minute.

If my kids are driving me nuts I can breathe for a minute instead of reacting in a way that feels terrible for all of us. I can thoughtfully respond and offer a natural consequence instead of blurting something out that doesn't make sense—and then being stuck with it.

I can go from chaos to calm in one minute, and I'm excited to share all of my techniques with you so you can have the same experience in your day-to-day life.

I believe that one-minute meditations are the glue that binds my days together so that moment to moment I am bringing my best self to the world.

Even my husband, who was a skeptic of meditation, now uses these meditations as a stress reliever in his job in the financial industry.

Let's face it. All hell can break loose at work, at home, or on the freeway in sixty seconds or less, so we must have tools to bring ourselves back to center and balance in just as short an amount of time.

The philosopher William James states, "The greatest weapon against stress is our ability to choose one thought over another." This is where awareness plays a huge role. We can't change anything in our life without first being aware that there is an issue. If you feel that stress is overtaking your life and the way you handle people and situations, then you have reached awareness, and you can begin to change. You are holding this book in your hands, so I believe you have taken the first huge step!

Chapter 3

What Can You Do?

A Perspective Shift to Encourage Consistency

> What you see depends not only on what you look *at*
> but also where you look *from*.
> —JAMES DEACON, HEALER AND AUTHOR

On my way to a speaking event in San Antonio, I had a mini melt-down. I was in an Uber on the way to the airport, and I realized that something in my life wasn't working.

I had read an article about a book on simplicity, and I went directly to Amazon to check it out. That book didn't feel like an energetic match, but another one called *Soulful Simplicity* by Courtney Carver jumped out at me. After perusing the reviews for a moment, I realized it was just what my soul was calling for.

I downloaded it mid-ride to the airport and read the entire flight and the few quiet hours I had to myself at the hotel before my event. It was quenching a thirst in me that I didn't even realize I had until that day.

The moment that I finished the last page, I grabbed my journal and frantically began pouring my heart onto the paper, documenting in detail everything about my life that needed to be revamped and simplified. The following excerpt is unedited and reflects exactly where I was in that moment.

I have come so far. I have done things in the past six years that make me feel really proud like:

- *Learning to meditate and creating beautiful self-care rituals*
- *Starting my mornings from a mindful, soul-centered place*
- *Learning how to handle stress so much better*
- *Becoming a more patient and connected mother*
- *Becoming more compassionate toward myself and others*
- *Learning to listen and connect with my intuition*
- *Embracing that I have so much to teach and give, and by sharing I can truly make a difference for other people*
- *Finding a career that fills me up and brings me huge amounts of joy*
- *Signing up for Kundalini Yoga teacher training*
- *Realizing that I need more time away from technology because as much as I enjoy it, it makes me feel disconnected from the people around me that I love and want to be present for*

Even with all this, something doesn't feel quite right. I don't know if I plateaued, or if it's time to take mindfulness to the next level in my life, but a few things happened which made me feel like I hit a "rock bottom" of sorts and heralded a wake-up call that I desperately need.

- *A friend asked me to have coffee and I told her we could in three weeks because that was my next available free hour during the week. She looked at me like I had two heads.*
- *I realized I couldn't have a lunch date with my husband for a month because I was so over-scheduled. A freaking month!*
- *I feel anxiety walking around my house because there seems to be a pile tucked away in almost every corner. The clutter is making me feel claustrophobic in my own home. I don't need to be on Hoarders, but it's a lot for me!*
- *I can't write my third book. I was extremely diligent about writing an hour a day for my first two books. It wasn't strict discipline in a way that felt crazy or overbearing, but rather so much passion and commitment surrounded them that I was able to tune a lot out and really focus. This time around I feel so distracted that I make every excuse not to write. Work travel, errands, calls, organizing all seem to come first. I absolutely cannot focus even though I am extremely excited about the material and topic, and it is stressing me out. I feel pulled in too many directions, over-scheduled, and worn out. I allot an hour a day on my schedule to write, but if I have to pee or I answer a phone call, I feel pressed for time and more anxiety sets in, which doesn't help the creative process! My writing time is always stacked right up against something else on both ends, so it feels like the clock is ticking and lots of pressure. If I go over by five minutes that means I am late for something else, like picking up my kids!*

- *When I look in my closet and medicine cabinet the first thought I have is, Where did all of this stuff come from? It makes me feel wasteful and kind of sad. Why am I accumulating so much stuff? Not to mention I even have duplicates of lots of makeup because I don't pay enough attention to what I already have so I keep buying the same colors. It's ridiculous.*
- *I feel like for the very first time I am not following my own best advice. I sometimes talk to clients, or reread parts of my own book, and think, I should be doing more of that!*

What I realize:

- *I am ready for change.*
- *I don't want to feel like important projects, especially writing my book or seeing clients, are so jam-packed in my day that I can't bring my very best energy to each one.*
- *I need more room to breathe, both in my home and in my calendar.*
- *I need even more time away from technology.*
- *A lot of my busy is in the name of self-care, but it's time to stop looking outside of myself for the resources to make me feel centered and do more of my own soul searching.*
- *I want to do an even better job being present with my kids. I am good, but I could always be better. This usually involves not looking at my phone and realizing that answering emails can wait. People aren't expecting a response in five seconds.*
- *I am buying to buy. Not all the time, but a lot. Even*

though I love trying new products and I love makeup and clothes, there isn't enough time to use everything I am accumulating. Here's a perfect example: I was dying for these amazing black loafers that were going to make me look chic and extremely pulled together. I spent a fortune, which is okay sometimes because quality is important, but as I think about it, I haven't been living in them like I thought I would. I have worn them exactly twice. They are sitting in a mass of shoes that were all supposed to make me feel pulled together and chic and most of them just sit there. I am not enjoying my things to the fullest because there are too many of them. This doesn't feel good anymore.

- *My writing time should not be pushed against carpool time. Mornings may be better this time around.*
- *I need to prioritize big time when it comes to my time, purchases, and what is filling me up. Why am I looking outside myself?*

And most importantly . . .

- *I am evolving and growing. What worked for me a few years ago may not work now. I am different. When I am not present with my kids it hurts my heart. I need more down time to feel centered, and I like more time alone than I used to. My job has changed because I travel more to speak (which I love), so this means my weeks may need to be structured differently. I need to think about how things are going to feel for me and my family instead of filling up every available hour, and booking things back to back. This used to work for me, but it doesn't anymore.*

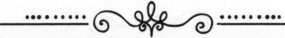

And it's okay. I want to embrace who I am now, realizing that I'm human, not superhuman. I can't be everything to everyone, and my relationship with myself and my family will always come first. I may not make everyone in my life happy all the time, but I will always show up to what I say "yes" to with my best energy and everything I've got.

Why *I want to declutter:*

- *I feel overwhelmed and over-scheduled.*
- *I feel guilty when I look at things that I don't use or wear.*
- *Clutter makes me anxious.*
- *I don't want to be wasteful. Other people can use and enjoy the things that I am not using.*
- *I want to create more space in my thoughts for creativity.*
- *I want to find even more joy in experiences with those that I love.*
- *More joy, connection, and time for people I love.*
- *I want to be a human being, not a human doing.*
- *I want to allow more authenticity to shine.*

What *I want to declutter:*

- *My drawers, closets, pantry, and coat closet.*
- *CDs and movies that haven't been used in years and years.*
- *I want to finish reading the stacks of books I have, and add new ones to a list.*
- *My calendar! It should feel more spacious.*

- *What we are holding onto in our attic spaces. This is probably the last priority though.*
- *What I say yes to, and when I choose to say no.*
- *I want to organize my recipes better and evaluate which cookbooks to keep and what is just taking up space crammed into my kitchen.*
- *I need to unsubscribe to the online publications that make me want to over-consume. Getting multiple newsletters every day with new products to try isn't helping me!*
- *So many appointments. What self-care beyond my own meditation, journaling, gratitude, energy work, and prayer do I want to prioritize? I don't have to work with every healer I love at the same time, and taking breaks is okay. I think I am kind of addicted.*

I understand that this will be a process. As I've always said when it comes to meditation, mindfulness, and other self-care practices, real change happens slowly, and I will never underestimate how much of an impact small changes have on my life.

I am not on a timeline, I am going to let my heart navigate this process.

I am looking at this process as the next phase in my evolution—one that puts the love I have for myself and the love I give to others at the forefront. I am not sure how this will all unfold exactly, and that's okay. Each baby step will be a gift that I give to myself and my loved ones.

This may look like one closet being de-cluttered, saying no to something that my heart isn't into, or taking an item off my to-do list. Some days I may do more, and some days I may do less.

I know that I am ready for change. I'm ready for the next

steps that will make me feel even more nourished, loved and loving, mindful, grateful, and content. What I hope to embrace fully on a heart and soul level is this:
> *I have enough. I do enough. I am enough.*

This is probably one of the most vulnerable things I have written and shared since my first book, *Hot Mess to Mindful Mom*, came out and I wrote the chapters on forgiveness and money. Those actually kept me up at night, and the night before it was released I vividly remember thinking, *OMG! People are actually going to read this!* I felt a little like I was standing on a street corner in my underwear, totally exposed.

Heart-Centered Social Media

When I first started teaching and writing I thought I had to appear like I had it all figured out. I only wanted to share what I was doing right, never what wasn't working in my life or things that felt hard. Why would someone want to learn from me or read what I have to say if I didn't do it perfectly myself?

Trying to be perfect doesn't make me real, and now I understand it's a turnoff because it isn't relatable. The truth is this: I work on all of the tools that I teach just as much as my clients. Day in and day out I am practicing being in the moment (and noticing when I'm not). I am making mistakes, learning lessons, and reminding myself to pause. This is why it's called a "practice." You are never done.

According to Ramani Durvasula, a professor at California State University, "Social media is basically social comparison on steroids." Even though it is human nature to compare ourselves to others, social media takes it to an altogether unhealthy level.

When I started sharing more of my own ups and downs, I really started to connect with the brave, amazing women who followed me on social media. The more authentic I became, the more engagement I had. Admitting that being present and fitting in self-care was sometimes a challenge in my busy life made me more relatable, and I relaxed and began having more fun on social media. We are all dealing with many of the same issues and challenges, me included.

I coined the phrase for myself, and I began telling people I practiced heart-centered social media. I no longer posted because I *had* to be super consistent, which had led me to sometimes slap up a post quickly and without much thought. Instead I became much more intentional and mindful. I began posting only when I felt inspired and truly had something worthwhile to share. It changed everything for me.

My Rockstar Client

I was doing a session with a rockstar client who lives in Bermuda. I love all my clients to death, but I will say that this lovely woman holds a special place in my heart because her follow-through is beyond amazing. I mean, she literally does everything we talk about. She has two precious little ones who get on our video calls. Her oldest loves to chat and would eat up our entire session if we let her! I have literally watched her son grow up—we began working together when she was pregnant, and now he's a full-on toddler. He melts my heart! She began as a weekly coaching client, and now we do a check-in once a month to keep her on track.

She has a very high-level job and is juggling feeling successful at work and at home, as so many moms are. We often talk about schedules and creating more flow in her home and calendar, how to

get out of work on time, as well as simple and efficient ways to sneak in as much self-care as possible.

I busted out an idea for her and loved it so much she had to give me a sec to write it down. It has since then become a mantra that I use for myself and every single person I work with.

"Never worry about what you can't do; only focus on what you *can* do!"

We were discussing meditation when this came up. Some days she simply can't devote the ten minutes to her daily seated practice, so I asked her, "Well, what can you do?"

There are so many opportunities to make a choice when it comes to meditation. Things like:

- Will I meditate today?
- Where will I meditate today?
- How long will I meditate today?

There are an equal amount of excuses when it comes to meditation too. Things like:

- I don't have time to meditate.
- I don't think it works for me.
- I'm not good at it.
- If I'm not going to do it long enough, I won't do it at all.

Meditation is one of the best places ever to practice self-compassion and let go of judgment. Day in and day out you have the opportunity to decide what direction you will go.

This has come up with so many clients over the years. They don't feel like their practice will be perfect or meet the expectations

that they have from scrolling social media of beautiful cushions, devoting long periods of time each day, and loose, flowy clothes. Meditation doesn't have to be any of those things. We are talking about meditation for the real world!

When my clients offer me excuses for why they can't meditate, I lovingly hold them accountable with this simple question, "What *can* you do?"

If you don't have twenty minutes to devote to your practice, do you have five? Do you have one?

If you didn't hit your cushion, can you meditate in your car in your parking space before you get out at work? Can you just breathe at a traffic light?

If you're stuck in a pencil skirt and heels at work, can you do a quick meditation in your office chair? Can you take one minute to plant your feet on the ground and breathe between tasks?

The mind will offer up excuses all day long if left unchecked. It's my job to see through my clients' excuses and then teach them how to see through the excuses themselves so they learn to ask the same questions when I'm not there.

Meditation offers us a chance to give up perfectionism and self-criticism. Don't let having a "perfect" meditation routine get in the way of actually having one at all.

I can't declutter and organize my entire life in one fell swoop, just as you can't expect to settle into your meditation practice overnight. Even on those days when mom life feels like a total shit show we can ask ourselves the important question, "What *can* I do?"

Chapter 4

Living with an Abundant Mentality

Feeling Lack or Abundance Is a Choice

Abundance is not something we acquire. It is something we tune into.

—WAYNE DYER, AUTHOR AND SPEAKER

I love the phrase "where attention goes, energy flows." I wrote a lot about the law of attraction in my second book, *Get the Most out of Motherhood*, so I'll just touch on it here briefly.

It's a universal fact that what you put your attention on gets bigger. Yup. Sweet and simple.

If you focus all your attention on negative thoughts or emotions, you will be living a pretty low vibe life; however, if you focus attention on positive emotions and thoughts like gratitude, then life will feel full and joyful.

It's not that we want to ignore feelings that are less than desirable—not at all. We want to process them, learn from them, and then move on from them.

This can manifest in so many areas of life—and *has* for me both personally and professionally, even in my social media habits.

I love social media because it allows me to connect with people and readers that I would ordinarily never know, and it can feel very inspiring to see what people I admire have to say. It is a fun way to keep in touch with family and people from my past, as well as new friends. In this day and age, it is also a great way to share what is going on in my family, and as a business owner it is a wonderful way to market my services and books.

Like anything, there can be downsides too. If I'm not careful, social media can be a black hole and a major time-suck. I could easily ignore my family and responsibilities for hours on end if I didn't keep myself in check. It is my aide in procrastination, and here's where the feelings of lack come in—I can find myself down a twisty road of judgment and comparison easily if I do not keep myself in check.

I hate actually admitting that, but I can't be the only one! Feelings of lack can creep up whether we are seeing pictures of someone's exciting vacation when we are sitting on the couch during spring break or witnessing an author's book launch via Instagram and contemplating that there're books more successful than mine. Major *yucks*!

I had to call myself out on these feelings of lack and bring more awareness to when they surfaced. I knew I needed to make some changes to feel more abundant around social media.

How I've made social media more heart-centered:

- I only go on social media Monday through Friday, so I am more present with my family on the weekends. No more getting sucked into the big, black hole during family time.
- I do my best not to go on social media when the kids get home from school until after dinner. Again, to be more present.

- I am more intentional about my posts. Instead of quickly slapping something up to maintain "consistency," I wait until I can construct a post of real value. This means I post a bit less often, but truly connect with my followers.
- I am more authentic and vulnerable. I don't just share what is going right in my life, but the struggles too.
- I focus less on how much my numbers are growing and more on how engaged my followers are.
- I monitor my time online each day. I try to be under two hours.

Now I enjoy my weekdays on social media, and I treasure my weekends off. I get excited to post because I am sharing from my heart more and more. If I ever notice feelings of lack, judgment, or comparison creep up, I immediately turn off my phone or computer and ask myself "Why? Where do I need to do a little soul-searching or work?"

Self-compassion is also key when these feeling arise. When I first became more aware of these feelings surfacing I thought, *What is wrong with me? Haven't I made more progress than this?* It can be eye-opening, but there is no going around an issue, only through.

I truly had some work to do around the abundance of time as well. I think many people do. We look at our calendars and to-do lists, and think, *There is just no way!*

Have these words ever come out of your mouth?

- I wish I had time!
- If only there was time . . .
- I'll never get this all done!
- I'm just *so* busy.

The truth is, there *is* time. The attitude we bring toward time, either lack or abundance, makes all the difference. If we believe there won't be enough time, there won't. We will be operating at a vibration of lack. Since like attracts like, if we feel lack, we will get more of it.

The days when I am in lack around time it seems like all of the traffic lights are red, salespeople are slower than normal, and I get held up at every train. Conversely, the days that I feel abundant and relaxed around time, traffic lights are green and errands happen quickly.

There are also other factors which I have found helpful in creating a more abundant mentality around time. They are . . .

My Attitude: Time isn't something to race or beat, it's my partner in getting things done. A bad attitude will usually lead to poor results in just about anything, including how much we get done in a given day.

Having Realistic Expectations of How Long Things Will Take: When I got honest around how long things take, and I began to prioritize what I could actually do in a day, my days began to flow in a new way.

Using Affirmations to Raise My Vibration: When I feel myself beginning to stress about getting things done, I will often use an affirmation to realign my energy back into a vibration of abundance. I will repeat it out loud or silently, depending where I am. After a few rounds I can feel my body settle and my energy and attitude shift. A few of my favorites are:

> *I get everything done with ease and grace.*
> *Time is my friend.*

I have enough time.
I flow through my day.
Time is on my side.
I am calm and relaxed.

I find that the more I focus on raising my vibration, the better my energy is and the more I get done. When I give myself ample time for self-care, and even to veg a bit, I am much more productive during my "get stuff done" time. I am not running errands wishing that I had time to meditate or journal. I get done what I need to for myself first, which leads me to feel better overall, allowing me to be more focused on the next set of tasks that I need to complete for either work or my family.

Meditation is a great place to investigate our feelings about time. If I had a dollar for every time someone told me, "I don't have time to meditate," I would be a *very* rich woman! Guess what? You do!

The first question I ask people is, "How much time do you spend on social media?" There are probably (most definitely) a few minutes that could be shaved off there!

My second question is usually, "Do you have one minute you could give to meditation?" When I tell people about one-minute meditations I get reactions like, "Oh, I could definitely do that!" or "I never thought of meditation like that!"

One-minute meditations are wonderful because they don't take much time, but add up to big change. Imagine what your life would feel like if you calmed yourself down every time you felt stressed. How would it feel to use typical downtime like waiting in line to create mindful minutes in your day? Would you be excited at the end of the day when you counted up your one-minute meditations and you racked up ten of them? Quick meditations are a great way to move from lack to abundance around having time to meditate.

Bringing awareness to your attitude around meditation and self-care can be extremely helpful in understanding if you need to make a change. What category do you fall into here?

When you have a lack mentality you may do the following:

- Tell yourself you don't have enough time to fit it in.
- Have a negative self-dialogue and tell yourself things like, "I suck at this" or "This can't be working."
- Feel resentment toward people that do a better job fitting it in.
- Feel jealous of people further on their path.
- Feel fear around making a change in your life.

When you have an abundant mentality you may do the following:

- Be willing to take a leap of faith and start a new routine.
- Believe there is enough time to fit in meditation and self-care.
- Understand that starting small is okay, as long as you start!
- Know that you are deserving of self-care.
- Trust that the Universe has your back and will conspire to help you succeed.

Huge shifts and change can occur when you are aware of your vibration and energy around situations in your life. Of course I invite you to bring your attention to meditation and self-care, but by no means should you limit it there. This same concept can be used when it comes to money, relationships, jobs, and anything else in your life.

It's funny (but not funny) that the week that I was working on this very chapter the Universe gave me two situations to work on around relationships—one that was mine, and one that was my son's.

I have a long-time friend that treats me like her personal Angie's List. I only hear from her when she needs something. I am always happy to share my many connections with people—in fact I love to because it helps my friends as well as the service providers I am recommending. For some reason though this time it rubbed me the wrong way. None of her texts ask how I am or even start with "hi." It's only about what she needs.

I called my friend to vent and explain that I am happy to share, but every once in a while it would be nice to connect about something else. I got it off my chest but immediately felt super yucky. I didn't like the feeling of raging on my friend, and I felt very low-vibe about the whole thing. I realized I was in lack around this.

I asked myself what a more abundant outlook on the situation would be, and right away I realized how grateful I felt that a friend knew she could count on me to help her. I was able to save her time and make her life easier, as well as get business for providers I think are wonderful and work really hard. All of a sudden I was in abundance around the situation and I felt so much better.

The very next day I was having breakfast with my boys and one of them complained about an annoying habit their friend had. This was a great opportunity to teach about lack and abundance.

I asked my son if his friend had more annoying habits or more great things about him. No surprise, he said great things. I used this as an opportunity to explain that everyone is annoying sometimes . . . even me, and even him. When we care about someone we have to accept all of them, even the things that occasionally get on our nerves.

We also have a choice to focus on the negative or the positive, and what we choose becomes our focus.

Are you in lack or abundance? What can you do to shift your energy if you need to? If you want ideas, keep reading. I will be sharing tools that you can use to shift your attention in one minute soon!

Chapter 5

Balance Is a Constant Recalibration

Failure Is a Thing of the Past

The two things in life you are in total control over
are your attitude and your effort.

—BILLY COX, AUTHOR AND PEAK PERFORMANCE STRATEGIST

One day I realized what my true definition of balance is. That was a *really* big day. It changed a lot for me.

So many moms, myself included at times, feel like a total failure. It seems like everyone else has their shit together and life seems to flow easier for them. This just isn't true!

Social media often gives a false impression of what someone's life is *really* like. By offering a well-curated taste of posts and pictures with the perfect filter, it's easier to come across as a supermom, fashionista, chef, and incredible organizer. Now, that's not to say that people aren't really, really good at all of this, but we all have off days!

I used to think that balance was something to achieve. I thought it was a destination, a place I would arrive at, and if I was a very good girl, stay at. This was the root of the problem. My expectations were *way* off.

Thanks to trial and error, I figured out that balance isn't a *place*, it's a *moment* in time. It's a moment that comes and goes, and it's up to me alone to realize when I've fallen out of balance and to recalibrate so I can get back.

Balance is a constant recalibration. When we fall out of alignment and balance we use a tool to get back as quickly as we can. Spoiler alert—you have thirty-five coming your way later in the book!

I'm going to share some lessons I've learned about balance along my journey.

Spiritual and Stressed Are Not Mutually Exclusive

I think there are some serious misconceptions out there when it comes to spirituality. I'll admit I had some at the beginning of my spiritual journey. Looking back, I get a big kick out of some of the crazy things I thought I was striving for. Oy!

Once I began meditating, becoming more mindful in my life, and prioritizing self-care, I didn't think I'd be stressed at all. Ever.

I knew that meditation was making me less reactive and more responsive, and I truly felt that, but I was waiting to never lose my patience or get frustrated and overwhelmed again. When I did occasionally lose my cool, I judged myself (and felt like others were judging me). Like I was a fraud instead of just being human! This is when I really came to terms for myself and began educating others about expectations.

We are all human. We are going to make mistakes, that is how we learn. We are going to lose our cool so we remember to use our tools. We are going to have off days for sure, we just hope for way fewer of them.

Awareness about What Makes Me Feel Good

I've grown so much in the past few years, so it's inevitable that I will have outgrown, or grown into, different things in my life.

One of the biggest things that I have outgrown is gossip. It just feels terrible now. If I participate I feel like I need to take a shower afterward.

I can remember when my kids were really little sitting around with a few friends talking about someone else. Why did I take part in something so mean-spirited?

According to the website Know Thyself, we gossip when we have low self-esteem, jealousy, or frustration, we want to appear more worthy, or we feel inferior. That pretty much sums up where I was at the time!

Psychology Today shares that anthropologists believe that throughout human history, gossip has been a way for us to bond with others. I think we can all agree there are better ways to bond.

I always tell my kids that happy people don't make others feel small; they build people up. If someone isn't being nice they may not be happy inside for some reason. We don't necessarily know what it is, but we can have compassion for them since someone isn't usually mean for no reason. This isn't to say we condone the behavior, and we should always stand up for ourselves and our friends, but it can give us a better understanding as to why they are behaving in a cruel manner.

When it comes to gossip I have made an across-the-board decision that, as a happy person, it is my honor to build people up, whether it is in front of their face or behind their back.

When I Blew Myself Off, I Paid the Price

There has been some trial and error around what it takes to keep me feeling optimal in my body, mind, and spirit.

- Once in a blue moon I have skipped my meditation and felt "off" all day. Daily meditation is totally non-negotiable.
- Getting a short second meditation in each day is amazing, but it doesn't happen 100 percent of the time. I consider it a bonus if it does, and I am striving for more consistency here.
- I notice a difference in my energy when I am doing Kundalini Yoga regularly. So much so that I became a teacher! I can't wait to make Kundalini more relatable and accessible, and teacher training was also a perfect way to keep me on track and consistent.
- I love journaling, but doing it a few times a week is enough for me. I really let my intuition guide me here.
- Energy management is non-negotiable. As an empath, I must clear and protect my energy daily and detach from anything I pick up from other people that doesn't serve me.
- Prayer has become second nature to me. I pray all day long!
- One-minute meditations, the point of this whole book, are my jam because they work. I mean, I *am* writing an entire book on the topic! I couldn't survive my days without these bursts of mindfulness that ground and center me throughout my day. Trust me, you will feel the same way!
- Connection with other people is essential to my well-being and balance. I have written before about being more introverted than I ever realized and not feeling totally comfortable in groups. However, I crave true connection and

conversation with like-minded souls and close friends. I also prioritize quality time with my husband and kids and need lots of hugs and eye contact with them every day.

- Connection to spirit is a literal Godsend in my life. I am only starting to open up about this, but I have been working with an amazing mentor to help me open my gifts for connecting with spirit. I feel without a doubt this is part of my path, and as one of my angels informed me one day, "Connection to spirit is my birthright." I do not think it is a coincidence that my entire spiritual journey began with a mediumship reading that the Universe literally pushed me into!

- There is something about my dogs that fills me up like nothing else can—in a future lifetime I hope I get to be a zoologist or a vet. Their presence and unconditional love is a true gift each day and I think my dogs make me a better person.

My Relationships Let Me Know Where I Was Emotionally

There was once a time when I would look outside myself for answers when something was wrong, but not anymore. I am done blaming other people for any unhappiness in my life, and if there are multiple areas in my life that seem to be suffering, then the undeniable common denominator is me. Maybe that is how I know I am truly, and finally, mature! I can now see with the trained eye of an artist what I need to work on and why. I don't have the ability to change other people or situations, but I can undoubtedly change my reaction to them.

If I am ever feeling disconnected from my husband, my kids, or friends, it is an obvious sign that something is off with me. I am usually ruminating about the past or worrying about the future, which means I am not where I should be: in the present moment.

I look at my kids and see how fast they are growing up. My oldest son towers over me, and is bound to overtake my husband too. Where is the time going? I don't want to look back and regret all of the energy that I put into situations that didn't serve me, toxic people, and energy vampires. I want my attention and focus to be on the joy in my life and connecting with people I love.

Fortunately, I can recover pretty quickly using all of the tools that I will be sharing with you shortly.

Reality vs. Dream Life

Life is perfectly imperfect. Every stage is just as it should be, whether it be a challenging one, or one where we feel like it is smooth sailing. The problem occurs when we have different expectations and feel disappointed with where we are.

Society can make us feel like if you aren't married by thirty and have two (and a half) kids, a house with a fenced-in yard, a nice car, and a fulfilling job that also allows you to have a neat and organized home and cook a healthy, Pinterest-worthy dinner each night, that you are failing.

Real life is messy, and hard, and complicated, and exciting, and fun, and full of lessons. There are times I have to remind myself, "This is your life. Be *in* it." I am not perfect at it, but I am learning to embrace the winding road because I learn from the twists and turns.

Where I am working on balance in my life:

Workouts

I used to feel like I failed any day that I didn't exercise. I set the expectation that for a day to be full and successful it must include a workout. I am much more in tune with my body these days, and sometimes I am tired and need more rest. Success around workouts is now measured by the week. I try to get in one or two weight sessions, one run, and a few walks with my dogs. It feels manageable and perfect for me.

Energy Management

As an empath I have to be cognizant of how much energy I am taking on from others because I can easily suck up anything around me. I have been studying energy for a few years and working with an expert to learn how to manage my own energy, protect myself from absorbing other people's, and clearing myself when I do. It has been an incredibly empowering journey, and I am now beginning to teach others how to manage their energy, which is thrilling for me.

Work/Mom Balance

I would be hard-pressed to find any mom, working or not, that doesn't ever feel guilt, but especially with working moms, it's constantly lurking.

There are times I have to travel for speaking events or am gone at night to do a workshop or see a client. I try to spread them out, but it is always hard to leave and miss anything with the kids.

This has made me so much more aware of how present I am with the boys when I am home. I try to stay off my phone between pickup after school until after dinner so I can focus on them and their needs, and I will give extra-long tuck-ins and snuggles as long as they will take them! I repeat to myself constantly the affirmation "present over perfect," because it reminds me that I won't ever be a perfect mom, but I can do my best to be a present one.

I do try to also think about what I am teaching my kids about independence, following your dreams, and sharing your passion and light with the world. I hope they remember that I helped make the world a better place for many, many people, more than they remember that one game I missed.

Pushing vs. Allowing

I have had ups and downs as an entrepreneur. It is imperative to have a sense of humor when revisiting the lows! When I go back and re-read some of the offers I put out when I was first in business, they alternatively crack me up and make me a bit sad. They are oozing with desperation. I can feel it when I read, and it makes me want to sage my computer—and myself.

When I first hung my shingle, I used to take note of what everyone around me in the self-help world was doing to be successful, and I thought I had to do the very same things. Instead of coming across as authentic and appealing, in retrospect my offers came across as forced. I was pushing too hard.

After much trial and error, I learned how to allow. I learned how to let my intuition guide me instead of comparing my efforts to others in my field. I let go of the word "should." In fact, if any sentence started with "I should be," then I knew it wasn't what my heart wanted. That meant I was in judgment or comparison of myself.

I worked with wonderful coaches along the way of building my business, and they taught me extremely valuable lessons, but I had to take a break to see what came out of my heart and felt authentic to me. The lines became very blurred between what they wanted me to do and what felt soul-centered.

Once I let my inner voice guide me in business, things began to flow more naturally and effortlessly. I stopped pushing and began allowing. I developed more trust and faith and let myself be guided to the right opportunities.

Listening to My Body and Spirit Each Morning

There are so many things I want to do in the morning because I love them all and they center and ground me for the day, but I don't have the luxury of three hours in the morning to get it all done.

If I had no responsibilities but myself, I would do the following every single day:

- Meditate
- Kundalini Yoga
- Journal
- Shamanic journeying
- Work with angel cards
- Stretch
- Write out affirmations
- Pray

It just simply isn't possible to do all of it every day in the hour that I allot myself before my family gets up. It took some processing for me to be okay with this, but when the alternative is getting up at 4:00 a.m. every day, I had to prioritize based on how I felt each day. Even though I am a get-out-of-bed-and-go person, I don't want to do it quite *that* early!

For a long time I was very all-or-nothing and super strict with myself. If I missed a day or part of my morning routine, I felt like I was a failure and not committed enough to my growth. It felt like I would somehow slide backward into old habits and patterns, when in reality it takes a lot more than that to undo the strides and growth.

Because there are so many practices that call to me, I decided the best way to choose what I was going to do each morning was to check in with my soul and see what it needed in the moment. Some mornings longer periods of silence call to me, and others more movement feels right so I do a Kundalini set. Occasionally there are days that journaling doesn't feel right, so I may do a Shamanic journey instead. I have given myself the gift of flexibility in my routines, which makes me feel less like I am checking off boxes and more like I am feeding my soul.

Alone Time vs. Social Time

I have become so much more of a homebody in the past few years. I used to be out and about all day long, filling every moment I was without kids with a coffee, lunch, workout, manicure, or shopping. Quiet wasn't my thing. Until it was.

I now crave solitude, along with plenty of time with my dogs. I could happily stay home all day long some days, not talk to anyone and only see my dogs! My day would be filled with snuggles, walks outside, writing, meditation, and reading on the couch if I had the time.

This is not to say that I don't equally love my days of seeing clients and connecting with friends, but now I crave it all. I have the physical, emotional, and spiritual need for both connection and quiet. Some days they are in equal measure, and others are more one-sided. The key I have discovered is listening to my soul and intuition to see what I need when, and to honor that.

I have also learned not to book my calendar to the brim or I will be miserable. I need more space in my days or I have an undercurrent of chaos which makes me feel off kilter. I have to fight off the urge to fit as much as I can into a day and instead plan ahead, knowing that if a networking call happens a week later the world will not fall apart. I cannot plan more than one social lunch a week or I don't have enough time for writing, and I truly enjoy the beautiful lunches I make the time to prepare for myself at home. I swear I could eat lentil or chickpea pasta with sautéed asparagus, zucchini, and broccoli topped with vegan pesto five days a week!

Social Media

My reason for being so open about sharing my personal pitfalls of being a newish entrepreneur is two-fold. The first is that I want to help other new entrepreneurs out there be true to themselves right from the start, instead of it taking approximately two years like it did for me. The other is that I get a huge kick out of myself when I look back at my journey. I mean, we have to have a sense of humor about this stuff and not take ourselves too seriously. I had the best of intentions, but my internal compass was just a bit off in the beginning. Figuring out social media has been a big part of my journey.

I adore social media and the way I feel inspired by others, as well as honored to have the opportunity to make a difference in people's lives with my own posts. That being said, as much as I love it, I love myself more when I take breaks from it, which is why I have set boundaries for myself.

My meditation and mindfulness practices have made me much more honest with myself when it comes to what's working and what needs improvement in my life. I could see that even with these positive changes I was constantly thinking "Would this make a good post?" as I was going about my day, even when I was trying to be present with my family. I was thinking in terms of social media all the time. I connected with my intuition and could feel that I was ready to take the next step. A whole day off each week.

I wanted to see what it felt like to have an entire day away from social media (and my phone, as much as possible). I wanted to see if

I felt more connected to my family and more present in all my activities. No surprise, I did.

I was so much more relaxed on Saturdays when I was "off." I chose Saturdays because it coincides with Shabbat, the Jewish day of rest. It felt like a nice tie in for me as a Jew—even though I am not extremely religious, it felt like a win/win.

To say I became more relaxed on Saturdays is an understatement. I wasn't thinking about posts or cataloging my life for others, I was simply living it. I was playing outside with my kids more, reading on the couch if I had downtime, or taking an extra walk with my dogs. Without mindless scrolling, I had a lot more time on my hands!

I felt so good on Saturdays, definitely more tranquil, more grounded, and more centered, that I decided I wanted my entire weekend to feel this way. I set the intention of taking #weekendsoff of social media altogether. Committing to myself in this way felt like a huge act of self-care and self-love. One of the biggest of my life.

Another upside to taking the weekends off of social media is that I can model better phone habits for my kids. Since I am engaged with them, they in turn spend less time on their phones, so it has a positive trickle-down effect. I definitely am more lenient with my boys on the weekends when it comes to time online, but I want them to understand how important limits and boundaries are.

I won't lie: sometimes I'm really tempted to hop on social media on the weekends. I have actually opened Instagram before and done a mental version of a hand slap, immediately turning it off. I genuinely like social media, I just like myself more when I have breaks from it, and that's what I have to remember in moments of temptation.

As an entrepreneur, author, and speaker, I build my business on social media, and that is okay. People won't magically know about my books if I am not out there, so my weeks are about building my brand and working online.

As a mom, wife, and friend, my job is to truly be in each moment with those I love, especially on the weekends. That is sacred family time, and I want to be as present as possible. #weekendsoff has allowed me to spend more time connecting with loved ones, and resting my body, mind, and spirit.

On Mondays I feel excited to see what has been happening in my online world, but by the time Friday night rolls around, I once again feel ready to say goodbye to social media for a few days. I'm ready to unplug from the world at large and plug into the life that is right in front of me. My life.

Ask yourself if you would benefit from a bit more time offline. If you aren't ready to take a whole weekend off, what baby step could you start with? Can you commit to one small change? Consistent changes lead to huge results. Don't underestimate how much small changes matter!

Chapter 6

Reprogram Your Thoughts

Self-Care Isn't Selfish

> If beating yourself up worked, you'd be rich, thin, and happy.
> Try loving yourself instead.
>
> —CHERYL RICHARDSON, AUTHOR AND SPEAKER

If you look up the word *selfish* you will find this definition: "lacking consideration for others."

I would be hard-pressed to find a mom that fits into that category. From the moment our kids are born into this world, and bless us with their presence in our lives, we are concerned with their well-being, happiness, and every bit of minutia connected to their day-to-day lives.

Children become an extension of our every thought, and days are planned around their needs. We shift into this pattern happily because of the joy they bring to our lives, but if we aren't careful we can get left behind in the shuffle of carpool, filling out forms,

and helping with homework. This is where overwhelm and exhaustion can creep into our lives between the cracks of smiles, love, and laughter. They are sneaky like that.

So many parents feel like life is going so fast, and before they know it their kids will be out of the house in college or on their own. I felt this way planning my oldest child's Bar Mitzvah.

There are many American-style traditions that take place at Bar Mitzvahs, and one is showing a video montage of your child's life. We had four sections in ours: Adam from birth to present day, our immediate family of four, extended family, and Adam with his friends. Video editing is not my strongest gift, so I had our DJ compile Adam's montage after I gave them all of the pictures that I had lovingly sorted through.

My reaction to watching the montage for the first time was so much stronger than I ever expected. I am an emotional and sensitive person, and I get teary at everything from television commercials to the Olympics to almost every athletic event my kids have. I knew I would cry a little, and I expected that. I needed a few tissues for even the process of gathering the photos!

What I didn't expect was to be a complete mess for an entire day. I didn't cry through the montage, I bawled. I didn't leave my house for the entire day, and I cried on and off for the eight hours that my kids were at school. I sobbed through the montage about twenty times that day. The emotion hit me like a ton of bricks.

Between viewings I processed emotions about how quickly life was moving. I asked myself tough questions like, "Am I doing a good enough job? Am I 'in it' enough? How can I improve as a mom?"

I didn't hide from the waves of feelings. I didn't sweep them under the rug by telling myself I was being ridiculous and too emotional. I let myself feel every single bit. I didn't berate myself for a moment. Instead I gave myself the time to be in the emotion, to process feelings about motherhood and myself. I didn't hide from the overwhelming combination of sadness, joy, and gratitude that I felt simultaneously.

I gave myself the day as a gift. I blew off every single thing on my to-do list, and wallowed, and then I felt better. I felt better because I didn't hide from my feelings, but instead confronted them head on. If I hadn't they would continue to creep into my thoughts and potentially break through at an inconvenient time. I wanted to enjoy Adam's weekend thoroughly, not be a bawling mess.

I woke up the next morning and it was a new day. I felt refreshed and blessed with a new level of presence and clarity which allowed me to soak up every sweet moment of my son's milestone. I also knew that some major self-care would be part of my emotional recovery. Crying for hours and hours is exhausting! I treated myself with kid gloves the following day by doing an extra-long meditation and Kundalini Yoga practice, gifting myself time to journal and to connect with a trusted friend about my feelings. Then once I felt stronger I went online to share my experience with my online community. I am glad I did because it sparked a lot of conversation about what it means to be a good mom. I try my best to be a good example for my kids, and sometimes that means forgiving myself for dropping the cape and just being human.

Over the years my parenting philosophy has really done a 180. My kids and their needs are always at the forefront of my mind, but what I need is evaluated in equal measure.

When my boys were younger I judged others who weren't trying to be supermoms. I thought they were selfish and lazy. Sad as it sounds, evaluating what other people did was high on my priority list. Looking back, it's easy to see why my kids had a mom that was overwhelmed, exhausted, and short-tempered. I wasted tons of my energy on comparison, feeling I needed to prove myself and my worth, and be "Supermom" to the outside world, instead of simply focusing on connecting with my kids and soaking up every moment of their early years.

Hindsight is twenty-twenty, and I can't change any of that now. My only choice is to beat myself up forever, or to garner all the lessons, improve, and share my insights and knowledge. I have obviously chosen the second path.

Looking back, the reduction in my level of anxiety and reactivity, coupled with the increase in my feelings of joy and confidence, in such a short time when I began to practice self-care is remarkable. It truly was quick. In a few short weeks of consistent practice, I began to feel myself blossom as a person and become more present as a mother. A little bit of time on myself each day bettered the life of my children by a lot. When I think about it that way it seems selfish not to practice more self-care! How good can we get? We can be so much more in every aspect of our lives than we ever realized.

As moms we need to flip the switch—maybe it's more selfish *not* to practice self-care.

I know these practices make me a better mom, but they also make me a better ME. They also make me a better friend, wife, coach, and speaker. I have come so far, and I am excited to see what my future holds. I will be the best surprise there is.

We can think in the context of motherhood, or we can evaluate our needs and hopes for ourselves, and there is nothing wrong with looking at life from that perspective. We were put on this earth to learn lessons and grow, and motherhood is just one part of that. We have needs too, and fitting them into the equation is essential to leading a satisfying life. Our kids will grow up and leave us one day.

They will always need us, and our love and support, but it won't be the day-to-day interaction and responsibility that we have now. If we haven't put any effort into ourselves and our growth up until that point, it can feel unbearable, and almost like we have been abandoned. There is no reason to wait until our kids leave home to begin working on ourselves. Don't wait five, ten, or eighteen years to be a priority in your own life.

We were given this one body, mind, and soul to act as our home for this lifetime. Don't we owe it to ourselves and the Universe to take care of it? There are many ways to do this, and everyone's needs around this are different:

- Time for journaling
- Reading a self-help book
- Time in nature
- Time to connect with loved ones
- Meditation
- Exercise
- Traditional talk therapy
- Energy healing
- Taking time to veg
- Mani/pedi
- Facial
- Massage

It's easy to compare to what others are doing, but self-care is totally individual, which is why "self" comes at the beginning of the phrase!

Create a judgment- and comparison-free zone. Let go of what others are doing and connect with your highest self so you can honor your needs. Have a "date it before you marry it" approach when it comes to self-care. Try something, and if it doesn't work for you, try something else.

You may be a person who likes to create one routine and stick with it, or you may crave more flexibility in your practices. There is no right or wrong, simply what works for you.

Check in with yourself now. What makes you feel most nourished? What makes you feel most connected to yourself? What makes you feel most relaxed and centered? Whatever the answer is, do more of that!

Chapter 7

Transition Times

One Missing Key to Success

Whether you think you can, or you think you can't—you're right.

—HENRY FORD

We carry the heavy burden of expectations from the outside world, and expectations that we put on ourselves, creating a (large) load to carry. We often internalize things like:

"I should be the perfect mom and never yell."

"I should only eat healthy food all the time and fit into all of my pre-pregnancy clothing."

"I should cook a perfectly balanced meal every night that we all sit down and eat as a family."

"I should . . ."

When we dream as a child about what life will be like as an adult, we think it will be peaceful and calm, money will flow plentifully, and we will be taking lots of vacations! This may be reality for a few people out there, but for many this is not how life feels.

One of my clients is a working mom and finds it very challenging to change hats throughout the day and to constantly switch from her responsibilities as a doctor to her responsibilities as a mom at the beginning and end of each day.

Life is busy, full, messy, fun, exciting, a little bit scary, and at times completely overwhelming. I think most moms would agree to all of these adjectives, but still wouldn't change a thing.

We are bombarded with pictures online of how other moms are handling life that look picture perfect, and I believe that our expectations get skewed for how life is supposed to feel and look.

Even though parts of each of my days are filled with meditation, Kundalini Yoga, prayer, and gratitude, I am balancing other parts with something cooking on three burners of the stove, both kids needing to be in different places at the same time, and most likely a dog barking. That's the messy part of life, but I have learned to embrace it all.

In *Get the Most out of Motherhood*, I shared that mindful parenting to me meant embracing each part of my day, and finding joy in each moment instead of feeling like I just need to "get through." More acceptance and joy filled my days when I stopped equating calm as my only measure of success. A household with two boys and two dogs and parents that work can be chaotic, and I've had to learn to embrace that or always feel unbalanced.

My meditation and mindfulness practices along with lots of prayer and gratitude are what fill me up and create the reserves in my being to handle a bit of chaos with more ease and grace. I don't freak out like I used to . . . instead I breathe, and I am not one typically made for chaos.

I always get a kick out of this: people assume that because of what I do, I don't have stress in my life. I hear things like, "You teach meditation and mindfulness? Your life must be *so* zen!" Thank goodness I have never heard this mid-sip, because I would probably have spit all over someone!

I have the same stress in my life as everyone else. I have two kids, two dogs, a household to run, work deadlines, client sessions, work travel, aging parents, and everything in between, just like you. What makes my life different is that I have a toolbox full of tools to help me manage and recover from stress so much faster, so that stress takes a backseat in my life, and joy has the steering wheel.

Learning to transition between tasks in my day has been one of the biggest game changers for me and my clients. I teach this to everyone I work with, whether they be forty or fourteen. This should be on everyone's radar if they want to get through the day without tearing out their hair.

We are so used to jumping from one task to another without a moment's pause to regroup, come back to center, or clear our energy if need be. What this means is that we are often taking stress or overwhelm from one situation right into another.

Imagine you are at work, and you have a heated discussion with a coworker because you disagree on how to move forward with a project. You realize you have a meeting so you storm off huffing and puffing, and muttering under your breath right into the conference room. You proceed to speak in a snippy tone and feel as though your entire day is shot. You race home to cook dinner and get the kids ready for soccer practice, all the while being short with your family, causing you to go to bed feeling guilty and like a failure as a mom.

That sounds like a horrible day!

What if the negativity was cut off right after the heated discussion with the coworker? Instead of going right into the next meeting, what if you took one minute in the bathroom, sat down on the toilet in a stall and did a quick body scan to release any tension that had built up in your shoulders and belly, followed by three nice, long, deep breaths to really help your nervous system chill?

Doing this allows you to walk into the conference room feeling more balanced and centered. Imagine then taking just one minute in your car in your driveway to count your breaths so that you can walk into your house having left work behind, ready to be Mom. How would that feel?

Don't Put Good Energy after Bad

It can feel impossible to turn things around in your day unless you make a conscious effort to do so. It doesn't just happen automatically. Instead we end up trying to put good energy after bad, which feels like swimming upstream.

What we put our attention on gets bigger, and our vibe either attracts what we want or don't want based on if we are feeling high vibe or low vibe. Crappy energy and feelings of fear, insecurity, judgment, overwhelm, shame, and comparison are obviously low vibe, so if we feel those types of feelings we need to do something to change our energy and our vibe so we can attract situations, people, and more feelings that are high vibe.

When to Use a Transition Tactic

Transitioning brings us back to the present moment so we can be fully engaged in whatever we are doing or experiencing in the moment. Whether it is at home, at work, or when we are doing something nice for ourselves, we want to be fully engaged. Transitioning can bring us greater feelings of peace and calm, and can increase our feelings of connection with others and ourselves. Here are some great situations to practice transitioning:

- When you change hats or transition your role in any way, whether it be leaving home to go to work, or leaving work to go home, you need to regroup. Getting out of the house in the morning can be stressful, so you don't want to take that energy into your workplace, and same goes for leaving the stress of work behind so you can walk in at the end of the day and be the mom that your kids need, and that makes you feel good.
- When you feel low-vibe and have any sort of feeling where you are just "off." You may be having a bad day, or you may have picked up some energy from another person around you. If so, give yourself a little regroup.
- When you are around someone low-vibe because energy can speak louder than words. Have you ever been with someone that complains all the time, is very judgmental, and has a negative opinion on everyone and everything, so much so you almost feel like you need a shower when you leave them? They are most likely pretty low-vibe. Reset each and every time after you see or talk to them!
- Between meetings at work is a great time to transition and re-center. Walk into each one feeling refreshed and open-minded.
- Between tasks as a volunteer because tensions can run high even at PTO meetings and volunteer organizations. People often feel tons of passion around what they are doing, which is wonderful, but can also lead to differing opinions and some drama.
- Before making a difficult phone call, to boost your confidence and feeling of ease. You may need another one after a difficult phone call to help you decompress and process with an open heart.

- Before and after any conversation you are nervous to have, because it will help you go into it feeling good and centered. I used to be a huge chicken when it came to conflict of any kind, but I've learned that speaking up for myself is necessary, and I can do it from a heart-centered place in as kind a way as possible. I typically need another minute of transition after the conversation because I most likely have some cortisol or adrenaline pumping in my body and I want to dissipate any feelings of stress as quickly as possible.
- Before a workout to feel more centered, since this is a special time for you to unwind.
- When you leave the kids to be social you want to be sure to dispel any feelings of mom-guilt. There is nothing wrong with leaving the kids for a bit! You need time with friends to feel connected, to laugh, to commiserate, and to enjoy a grown-up meal.
- Before a date night or spending time alone with your spouse, because this is sacred time for both of you. Try not to take the stress of the day into this time, and instead make each other laugh, and remember why you fell in love!
- Any self-care activity to feel more present, because what is worse than getting to the end of a massage or pedicure and feeling like you missed it because your mind was somewhere else?

How to Transition: Use any of the One-Minute Meditations from the next section!

Section 2

One-Minute Meditations and Practices

Get Ready to Change Your Life!

Between stimulus and response, there is a space. In that space is our power
to choose our response. In our response lies our growth and freedom.

—VICTOR FRANKL

When I was a child, I had temper tantrums. Big temper tantrums.
My parents decided they would try to get me to stop by showing
me how ridiculous I looked when I had them, so in the midst of a
temper tantrum at dinner everyone in my family stood up and cop-
ied me. They stamped their feet and yelled, and I will never forget
what it looked like. They looked like brats, and even then I understood what it meant that they were being my mirrors. As a little
girl, nobody taught me coping mechanisms for stress, frustration,
or overwhelm. I wonder if I would have had as many tantrums if I
actually had tools to deal with my feelings.

It's embarrassing to admit, but there was one time that I had a complete temper tantrum as an adult, reminiscent of the ones I used to have as a kid.

My son decided without asking me to log on to my new laptop. He thought he could guess my password, but he ended up locking me out of my computer, and when I finally could log back on, everything I had been working on was gone. Of course this was the week of a huge presentation, and I freaked with a capital F. I was not only crying, I was howling. I scared myself.

At one point my husband crept downstairs and asked if there was anything he could do. I looked at him with tears streaming down my face and I told him, "I know what tools to use, but I don't want to use them. I just want to cry."

This was a mistake. When I finally stopped crying I felt hungover, exhausted, and depleted. I was also so embarrassed that my kids saw me like that. I ended up doing a one-minute meditation, and once I calmed down I was able to figure out a solution for how to find my presentation on the computer. The reptilian freak-out part of my brain couldn't do it, but my calm frontal lobe could.

I promised myself that I would always use my tools going forward and acknowledged this as a not-so-gentle reminder that when my body is calm, my brain can think.

One-minute meditations have the ability to change your life, but tools only work if you use them! The goal of these practices is to find more peace in everyday life, to be more present, and more connected to those we love, and more connected to ourselves. The more you use one-minute meditations the more you crave them, because they work. They can bring you from chaos to calm in one minute or less. I don't know many other things that can that are actually good for you!

It is essential to practice using meditations before you feel stressed, so that in the moment of stress, when you need one to calm down, they feel natural.

Practice when you wake up, before bed, while you are nursing your baby, or cooking dinner. Practice in line at the grocery store, at a traffic light, or in the shower—there is no wrong time to use one. So let's dive in!

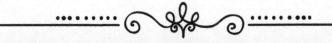

Meditations and Practices

Meditation #1:

Sigh It Out

It's crazy to think about, but most humans can live up to three weeks without food and three days without water, but only three minutes without oxygen. This makes it pretty clear that our breath is the key to our survival. Ancient yogis also claim that it is the key to vitality, talking a lot about prana, our life force energy, which we bring into our body with our breath.

As important as our breath is for sustaining life, many people don't realize that there are different ways you can breathe—and the style and pace of your breath can have a powerful impact on the state of your body and mind.

Shallow breathing doesn't give our bodies enough oxygen to function properly. When your breath is consistently shallow, stagnant air, residue, and pollutants can accumulate in the lungs, which can lead to low energy and toxic buildup. Deep breathing, on the other hand, supports healthier lungs, ensures that oxygen moves through the blood and all cells, detoxifying, energizing, and nourishing every part of your body along the way.

Our exhales ground and stabilize us. This is important to understand so that your breath can work for you in different situations when you are needing specific results. The easiest way to think about this is:

Longer exhales = calmer body and mind

Exhale to chill

When you're feeling stressed, anxious, frustrated, scattered, or overwhelmed, focusing on the exhale will help neutralize those feelings and settle both the mind and body. When we elongate our exhale, we are stimulating our parasympathetic nervous system.

I don't want to get too technical, but it can be very helpful to understand a bit about how your body works when it comes to stress and your breath. It becomes the "why" when thinking about your breath, and when it makes sense to you, you are more likely to use the tool of elongating your exhale.

There are two branches of the autonomic nervous system that regulate bodily functions associated with the heart, lungs, circulatory system, and glands. These are involuntary actions that your body does without you having to think about them. You don't think about your heart pumping blood, or your food digesting, it just happens. Thank goodness! The two branches are called sympathetic and parasympathetic.

The sympathetic system helps the body "gear up" when needed, accelerating the heart rate, raising blood pressure, and increasing tension in the large skeletal muscles. It also activates the stress response, or fight-or-flight response. When you feel stress, muscle blood flow is increased, pupils dilate, and perspiration increases. This is all happening so that your body can perform under pressure. Will you fight or flee?

The parasympathetic system does the opposite—decreasing your heart rate, lowering your blood pressure, and releasing muscular tension. This activates the rest-and-digest response where your body is operating at an optimal level. Your digestive system is in full swing and you feel calm and centered.

Inhalation stimulates the sympathetic system, and exhalation stimulates the parasympathetic system. When we are under pressure and thinking stressful thoughts, we often make ourselves tighter and more tense by inhaling longer than we're exhaling. Have you ever seen people under stress try to take deep breaths but they are really just raising their shoulders up? They are actually stressing their bodies out more! Just for kicks, try it now. Raise your shoulders up as you take a few powerful breaths. Do you feel more stressed or relaxed?

The remedy is straightforward and accessible: lengthen the exhalation—in fact, make it twice as long as the inhalation. Sustain this breath pattern for a minute and notice how your heart rate slows, your blood pressure drops, and your muscles begin to relax. Emphasizing your exhales also allows your lungs to discard toxins and carbon dioxide, leaving more room for fresh oxygen as you inhale.

It is important to fill your navel and chest as you breathe. The easiest way to know you are doing this is by feeling your belly rise and fall as you breathe. A teacher once used a great analogy: when you fill a pitcher, the water goes into the bottom first. Think of the air going into your belly as filling the bottom of that pitcher.

Have you ever noticed that when you feel really relaxed you sigh? That is a natural elongated exhale. You probably never thought of it that way. Your body is so smart! A good example of the relaxation response is getting a massage. My very favorite is reflexology, when just my feet get rubbed. Every time I sit in that chair and begin

to unwind, I sigh. This longer exhale helps my body relax and for accumulated stress to leave my body.

As much as I would *love* to be getting reflexology every single time I feel stress or overwhelm, that plan doesn't fit into my working mom life—or my budget! Fortunately, there are simple things we can do on our own, like a one-minute meditation where we elongate our exhales to help us in moments when we feel inundated by life, like making our exhale longer than our inhale.

It is important to be mindful of your capacity when you are setting the length of your inhale and exhale. Everyone's comfort level is different. I don't have a huge lung capacity, so I can't compare myself to someone that does. This is very personal, and you must listen to your body and do what is right for you. I call this finding your "comfortable edge." You want to push yourself to a place where you still feel comfortable and safe. Respect your body and its signals. If you extend your exhalation farther than your capacity allows, your body will go into survival mode and will want to gasp on the next inhalation. You'll need to shorten your next breath slightly in order to compensate. Your breaths should be smooth and you should transition from inhale to exhale and back to inhale with ease.

You have many options here. You can have an exhale one beat longer than your inhale, or you can double the length of your exhale. Try it a few ways and mix it up. See what you feel comfortable doing and notice when your body feels the most relaxed. Here are some examples:

- Inhale for two counts, exhale for three counts
- Inhale for two counts, exhale for four counts
- Inhale for three counts, exhale for four counts
- Inhale for three counts, exhale for six counts

Put it to work

- Sit comfortably, allowing your body to be comfortable yet alert. Set a timer for one minute, or two or three if you have more time.
- Focus on the rise and fall of your belly as you slow down your breath.
- Start to extend your exhale to twice as long as your inhale (or whatever count works for you).
- Notice how your mind calms down as you slow down your breath and focus on your exhales.

Meditation #2

Counting with Your Fingers

If I had a dollar for every time I heard someone say "I can't meditate because my mind wanders too much," or "I can't clear my mind," I'd be filthy rich! There are so many misconceptions about meditation and I wish I could take out a billboard on every corner in America to clear them up.

Meditation is about calming your nervous system and helping your mind to focus on one thing at a time, with an overall point of having a better life. What good is doing anything if it doesn't affect your life in a positive way? If you practice focusing on one thing in meditation, then you get better at focusing on one thing outside of meditation, for example your loved ones when they are talking to you. Instead of your mind wandering to work, or your grocery list, you are fully present and connecting. Trust me, people can tell when you are really paying attention, especially your kids!

Counting your breaths in meditation is a great way to maintain focus, but I have developed a way to supercharge this focus in also incorporating your fingers into the mix. Your breath is always with you, as are your hands, so this is a perfect one-minute meditation on the go!

1. Sit comfortably with your legs crossed or feet flat on the floor.

2. Maintain an upright posture. Feel your sits bones connect with the cushion or chair. Elongate your spine by reaching your crown toward the sky, and give your chin a very slight tuck.

3. Place your hands on your thighs and let them rest gently. No need to tense your hands.

4. As you take a comfortable inhale, silently think "one" and place all of your awareness on the tip of your left pinky. You can press your finger tip into your thigh gently if you want, but it is much more about simply using your awareness.

5. As you exhale, silently think "two" and place all of your awareness on your left ring finger and continue this pattern until you reach "ten" and the pinky on your right hand. It looks like this:

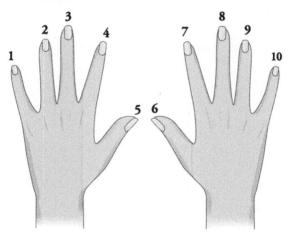

6. Repeat the cycle starting with your right pinky and work your way back to your left pinky.

In one minute, you can do approximately three cycles, but it depends on the length of comfortable inhales and exhales for you. There is no right or wrong, just maintain a pace that feels right to you and don't rush it.

If during this minute you notice your mind wandering, which it very well may, simply start over at "one." If you lose count, simply start over. This isn't a test, and you don't fail if you have to start over. We are building our focus and concentration muscles each time we do it. You get an A every time you sit!

Meditation #3

Body Scan

Release all your tension

When I feel stress, I immediately feel my shoulders tense. You too? You may also feel your tummy tighten or your hands clench. This is our body talking to us. I imagine mine is saying something like, "Ali, you are totally stressed in this moment. You are human, so it's normal, but you know you don't have to stay here. You have tools to help!"

When I feel stress in my body, I know it's a perfect time to do a body scan. Focusing on each part of my body and sending prana, breath or life force energy, there helps me to release tension and come back to center rather quickly, in about one minute.

If you have more time it is always wonderful to luxuriate in the experience, and you can take more than sixty seconds, but for the purposes of this book, we are going to do a body scan in one minute. You can do this at a traffic light, as a stressful meeting is kicking off, or before bed to let go of any tension that built up in your body during the day. When I do this and relax my body before bed, I can usually fall asleep faster.

Doing a body scan is simple—start at your head and work your way toward your toes. As you run through each body part you simply focus on relaxing that part of you. You will spend approximately three seconds on each major body part and you can get through your body in one minute. Here's how:

1. Use your position of choice based on where you are and the situation. You may sit up or lay down for a body scan.
2. Close your eyes and take a nice long deep breath.
3. Spend approximately three seconds on each of the following body parts:
   - Scalp
   - Forehead
   - Eyes
   - Cheeks
   - Jaw
   - Mouth
   - Shoulders
   - Left arm
   - Right arm
   - Left hand
   - Right hand
   - Chest
   - Belly
   - Hips
   - Right leg
   - Left leg
   - Right foot
   - Left foot
4. Take a nice deep breath in and out, and if your eyes are closed, open them.

The great thing about a body scan is that you cannot mess up. If you miss a body part, it's no big deal. Your body will 100 percent be more relaxed if you hit most of them. This is a low-pressure tool.

It's interesting to see where you are holding tension. I never thought of my cheeks as a place that I would need to relax, but it's amazing how much tension I am always holding in them! Keep an open mind, and let your body do its thing.

I also like to use a quick body scan before I eat. I notice that if I am anxious at all before I begin eating, that I eat really fast. I may not even realize what feelings I am holding in my body at the time, so before I begin a meal I do a version of a body scan where I take a nice deep breath and check in with my body to see if I am holding tension in any of my typical places. I don't do a complete body scan like the one above, instead I really hone in on how my body is feeling in that moment. If I notice tension in my shoulders, chest, or belly, I breathe into it and feel my body relax. Then I am ready to eat my meal from a calm place, at a peaceful pace.

Kids also love body scans. My kids ask for them before bed, and I always remind them to calm their bodies on test days. As the teacher is passing out the test, I tell them to be sure their bodies feel calm, because when our bodies are calm, our brains can think better!

Meditation #4

Gratitude Made Easy

What you focus on gets bigger

One of my favorite quotes about gratitude is from Albert Einstein, "There are only two ways to live: one is as though nothing is a miracle. The other is as though everything is."

Practicing gratitude can help you feel more alert and enthusiastic, have more determination, feel more optimistic, and have higher energy levels and sleep better. You may also experience fewer depressed thoughts, less stress, worry, and anxiety, and make more progress toward attaining your personal goals. Sign me up!

Focus on the rainbows

In the words of David Steindl-Rast, a Benedictine monk, "The root of joy is gratefulness . . . It is not joy that makes us grateful; it is gratitude that makes us joyful." The more we practice gratitude, the easier we can ride the waves of life. Yes, we need to process all emotions, whether comfortable or not, but we take responsibility for where we dwell. Do we stay rooted in the negative, or do we focus on the positive aspects of our lives? We see more good, and more joy. We notice the rain but we focus on the rainbows.

Dr. Christina Hibbert writes that gratitude can reduce negative emotions because feelings like anger, bitterness, and resentment are incompatible with gratitude. You literally can't feel both at the same time. So, if we cultivate more gratitude, we feel less negativity.

It can take practice to make the mindset shift in tough moments, but the more we put into this new way of thinking, the more joyful life feels. Here's a real-life mom example . . .

We all have strengths and weaknesses as parents, and parts that jazz us up more than others. Homework and studying are not the parts that light my fire. After dinner I am often tired, and I want to curl up with my own book while my kids are studying, but they want me to test them. This request could bring tears to my eyes some nights if I didn't infuse gratitude into the situation. I tell myself that they aren't going to need me like this forever, and I don't want to wish a moment of it away. So when I hear that inevitable, "Mom, will you test me?!" I say a silent "thank you" and I get a warm fuzzy feeling instead of wanting to scream, "I'm off duty for the next hour!"

Learn to see the good

Learning to see the good in your life even when hard times come is a powerful coping strategy that also takes practice. This happens when we acknowledge the lessons life is bestowing upon us and appreciate all the growth accompanying them.

It takes stretching our gratitude muscles on a daily basis so that we can count on them working in times of stress or overwhelm. I have a favorite way to practice gratitude that makes it feel easy and seamless in your day.

For about a year I kept a gratitude journal, but it began to feel like another "to do" on my already long list. I would forget half the

time, and then feel badly. I needed a way to make this important practice easier.

As a meditation teacher, I know that we have more success with incorporating a new habit if we attach it to something that we already do. So I asked myself, "What do I do every day?" and the first thing I thought of is brush my teeth. Yup. Twice.

I put an index card that simply says "Gratitude" next to my bathroom mirror near where my toothbrush patiently waits in a mason jar morning and evening. Every time I brush my teeth I glance at the card, and it reminds me to think of a few things I am grateful for while I brush. This way I am beginning and ending each day with gratitude. No journal, no pen, no pressure.

I found success with this tool, and so many of my clients have as well. It makes practicing gratitude and reaping the benefits a breeze.

Be a better parent

When you're able to cope better with life's ups and downs and find more joy and meaning in life, you will be a better parent. This translates to recognizing the good in your children, being able to express it to them, and in turn helping improve their self-worth, health, and happiness too. Gratitude is a cycle that allows us to feel good and pay it forward to those we love the most.

Gratitude glasses

A leading gratitude researcher, Robert Emmons, has defined gratitude as "a felt sense of wonder, thankfulness, and appreciation for life." Imagine how life unfolds in the most beautiful ways when we see our experiences and relationships through a lens of gratitude.

This reminds me of a beautiful message that I received in meditation one day. I was putting out to the Universe a question that had

been weighing on me a lot. I am sure I am not the only one in the world who wonders why, when I have done so much work around compassion and forgiveness, can certain people still trigger me so badly. It's almost like I want to throw my hands up and scream, "I processed this already! How can this still bother me?!"

This isn't the first time I have thought about this, how the same feeling can present itself to you again and again because there is a little bit more work to do around it, just like when you keep making the same mistake over and over until you finally learn your lesson. Then, when you finally gain enough awareness to acknowledge your stubborn pattern and change, the Universe moves you onto another lesson.

But back to the glasses.

I received a beautiful response, "See the world through rose-colored glasses. Everything will not feel or look perfect all the time, but you can see it all through the lens of love. When someone triggers you, or a situation feels hard, imagine putting your rose-colored glasses on and seeing again, but seeing from your heart with love."

What if we had gratitude glasses, and we were able to see our days through a lens of appreciation and wonder? What if birds singing in the tree outside our window wasn't just a random occurrence, but we viewed it as an event orchestrated by nature to bring us joy? How good would life feel then?

Use gratitude in moments of stress

Gratitude can easily be used in moments of stress as a one-minute meditation. Practicing a bit each day with our gratitude card makes it easier to use it as a tool when we need it. Gratitude can be used to refocus your attention in the face of overwhelm and frustration. It creates an energetic shift that allows us to stop focusing on negativity and shift into feeling more positive.

This can be as simple as thinking of three things you are grateful for, or as involved as journaling on the lesson you learned in a situation and why you are grateful you can move forward in your life with this newfound wisdom.

How can you stretch your gratitude muscles a bit each day? How can you use gratitude in the moment of stress? Remember, small acts lead to big change.

Meditation #5

Use Your Senses

We have them all for a reason

There are two types of distractions: **sensory distractions** are things happening around you, and **emotional distractions** are from your inner dialogue, and thoughts about things happening in your life. This is the chatter we hear in our head all day long. I believe author and actress Mindy Kaling calls it her "itty bitty shitty committee." I can't think of a better name for the negative chatter we hear seventy percent of the time!

It's sad when you think about it, we really spend most of our time beating ourselves up. Fortunately, the more we are aware of this, the faster we can change. For a long time, I would notice my "itty bitty shitty committee" and literally say out loud "Get lost! You are not invited into my day!" The more I did this, the less it showed up. Goodbye to at least most of the judgment and insecurity. The chatter of our own mind is the most distracting thing in the world.

When I notice thoughts or feelings creeping in that don't feel productive or nourishing, I aim to catch them as soon as possible, and use a tool to come back to a good place in my mind where I feel calm and centered. It always works to go to my "safe place."

Everyone has a "safe place," and a mental vacation to get there is always available to us. This exercise is best done with your eyes closed, so save it for a time and place that this is possible. Here's how you do it:

1. Sit comfortably or lie down.
2. Choose a place from your memory that you love. It could be from a favorite vacation, a favorite park, or anywhere that you feel relaxed. It's best for it to be in nature. I always use a beautiful beach in the Caribbean that I visited because a beach with clear blue water is my happy place.
3. Imagine in your mind's eye that you are in this place. Really let yourself feel it.
4. Use your senses to help you.
   • What do you see?
   • What do you hear?
   • What do you smell?
   • What can you touch?
   • What can you taste?
5. Give yourself a full minute, or more if you have it, to enjoy your treasured "safe place."
6. When you feel ready, slowly open your eyes.

Kids love using their "safe place" as much as adults. It's great before bed, before a test, or any time they are just in a bad mood, because nobody can be in a good mood all the time.

I tell my kids that everyone is entitled to be in a bad mood occasionally. It happens. We don't want to ignore our feelings, but we can't bring everyone around us down. If they are in a bad mood

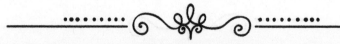

they can still be polite and kind to the family, or they are welcome to retire to their room to chill until they feel better. This would be a perfect time for them to visit their safe place.

Meditation #6

Essential Oils

Let nature be your mindfulness ally

I am by no means an essential oil queen, but I dabble, and do truly love using them. I appreciate the ritual of them, and the way they make me more mindful and present. Oils enhance my meditation practice and my desire to appreciate small moments during the day. There are also many health benefits to using them.

I always recommend using a therapeutic or medical grade oil that is 100 percent plant derived with no additional processing, preservatives, or other ingredients. You just want the oil.

Essential oils can help with things like:

- Better sleep
- Cleaning your home
- Opening your airways
- Soothing aches
- Aiding digestion
- Helping you relax
- Enhancing the flavor of food

I do love oils for all of these reasons, but I especially love them for the way they make me feel. They can either calm me or energize me based on which I use.

According to information from doTerra, the brand of oils that I use, our brains are designed to use aroma to soothe and protect themselves. As we inhale an essential oil, the aroma meets our brain in the olfactory bulb (also known as the "emotional brain") and triggers a series of chemicals. For example, lavender triggers serotonin, which has a calming and relaxing effect on the mind and body.

There are multiple uses for many of the oils, and here are a few of my favorite ways to use them:

- I use lavender when I meditate or on my feet before bed—the pores in your feet are larger, so this seeps into your bloodstream and works quickly to help you fall asleep. I also like to put one drop on my pillowcase to smell as I go to sleep. It's always nice to smell if I turn over in the middle of the night because the smell really lasts.
- I love to put a few drops of lemon in my water to help detoxify. It also makes the best homemade knockoff for Goo Gone.
- Lemongrass is one of my favorite smells. I add it to my unscented body lotion.
- I take salt baths with bergamot, which helps to soothe anxiety, ease sadness, and let go of what no longer serves you.
- I *love* the smell of the doTerra OnGuard immunity blend. I use the foaming hand soap and all-purpose cleaner. I clean my counters all the time just so I can smell it! I also diffuse it a ton in the winter in the kitchen and my kids' rooms.
- When I am cooking something smelly, like fish, I diffuse lemon and purify in my kitchen to get rid of the smell.

- I call peppermint "my coffee" because when I put a drop or two on the back of my neck, it totally wakes me up. I also put a drop on my tongue as a breath freshener.
- Neroli is a muscle relaxer, and I often rub it on my feet before I go to bed.
- I add frankincense to face products because it is supposed to help with wrinkles.

If you are looking to get started with oils, here are a few guidelines to get you going. I will recommend starting slow, and I say this from experience. If you buy too many oils at once it can become totally overwhelming and you may not end up using any of them. That's what happened to me. I got a bunch to start, and then I got confused and couldn't deal. I put them all in a cabinet for a few months and ignored them. I began to take one out at a time and get familiar with it. First I took out peppermint, then lemon, and then lavender, and began using those three until I felt comfortable. Then I slowly added oils to my counter and began using them on the regular.

- Calming oils: lavender, ylang ylang, geranium, vetiver, frankincense, melissa
- Invigorating oils: wintergreen, eucalyptus, peppermint, citrus oils
- Uplifting oils: lemon, orange, peppermint, bergamot, geranium, melissa
- Relaxing oils: lavender, roman chamomile, geranium, ylang ylang
- Stimulating oils: peppermint, eucalyptus, orange, grapefruit, rosemary, basil

When using oils, you can inhale them, diffuse them, or apply them topically. A few oils can also be ingested. Just be sure you know which ones are appropriate to ingest or apply to the skin. Since the oil comes directly from the plant, I use the rule of thumb that if I actually eat it in my diet I can ingest it, like lemon, orange, oregano, peppermint—but always check first!

There are many blends of oils, and my very favorite is called Balance. It has spruce, ho wood, frankincense, blue tansy, and blue chamomile.

As a one-minute meditation to help me regroup during the day, I will put a drop or two of Balance on my wrists. I rub them together and hold my wrists in front of my nose and inhale deeply. I take a few calming breaths like this and I notice my body begin to relax. Then I rub my wrists on my neck to distribute the scent. It's pretty heavenly.

Meditation #7

Drink Your Way to Calm

I have never been a coffee drinker, but I am a self-proclaimed tea junkie. I love the ritual of making tea as much as I love the taste. Whether it be mint, Earl Grey, or my beloved chai, I savor every sip.

When I am feeling stressed or overwhelmed, especially during a work day, I will often take a break from what I am doing to make a cup of tea. It helps to shift my attention away from worry, back into the present moment.

The process begins with picking my mug. I have a few favorites for sure. A long-time client gave me one that I love that says "meditation over medication." I bought one that says "You Rock" on a trip to New York City when I attended the very first Spirit Junkie Masterclass with Gabby Bernstein, and my very favorite one says "Karma is only a bitch if you are." I actually bought that one as a gift for a friend, but once I got it home I couldn't part with it, and I gave my friend something else. Sorry, Sarah! My newest addition is a travel mug with the chakras listed on it. That mug makes me so happy as I'm driving the kids to school in the mornings. It's really the little things!

I am sensitive to caffeine, therefore I typically stick to only

herbal blends after noon, so I don't have trouble falling asleep at night. I'm kind of paranoid about it!

Once I pick my mug and blend of tea, I set about the process of making it. My favorite kitchen gadget is my milk steamer. Years ago, I used to microwave my nut milk for tea, which makes me cringe to think about now. I am not snobby when it comes to most things, but I am glad my college friend set me straight about five years ago. I was visiting her in LA, and I set about making my tea in the morning. When I told her I would just put my milk in the microwave, she was like, "Not in my house!" Her husband is a majorly acclaimed chef, so they had the most pimped-out kitchen ever. I'd never even seen a milk steamer before, but I was hooked. I am pretty sure I ordered it on Amazon from the airport!

Taking the extra step to steam my milk has become a way of telling myself that I am worth the extra two minutes to make my tea even yummier. I love nut milk, usually almond or cashew, in my tea, and when I pour in the frothy yumminess it feels decadent. These tiny incremental up-levels can make life feel so nice.

Once my tea is made I truly savor the first few sips, usually with my eyes closed standing in my kitchen. Then I will decide if I want to enjoy the rest of my mug outside, sitting on the floor with my dogs, or back at my computer. Going back to work with tea in my hands can give me the boost I need and a fresh outlook.

Part of what feels so good about making and drinking tea for me is the ritual aspect of it. It makes me slow down and savor each step of the process so that I am truly in the present moment. Here's a ritual that makes me feel at ease:

1. Select your mug.
2. Choose which tea you will make.

3. Gather your supplies, such as milk, nut milk, honey, lemon, maple syrup, or sugar.
4. Brew your tea and add all your yummies to it.
5. Sit down comfortably.
6. Hold the mug in your hands and feel its warmth.
7. Take three nice, long, deep breaths as you hold the mug before you sip.
8. Feel yourself connect to the present moment.
9. Smell your tea and think of how you would describe its scent to someone else.
10. Take a sip slowly and hold the tea in your mouth for a moment and think about how you would describe its taste.
11. Sip the rest of your mug as slowly as you want and feel your body relax with each sip.

I thought it would be fun to share a few of my favorite tea recipes. I hope you enjoy them!

Ali's Chai

This chai is made with Blue Lotus brand chai and Vital Proteins collagen. You can find these in my Amazon store with all my favorite self-care products at www.amazon.com/shop/hotmesstomindfulmom.

    2 spoons (spoon comes in tin) of chai
    3/4 cup milk or nut milk of choice, warmed in steamer
    3/4 cup hot filtered water
    1 scoop vital proteins collagen powder
    Maple syrup to taste

Put all ingredients in a high-speed blender and drink right away. (My suggested Blue Lotus brand works this way—if your chai requires steeping instead, do so before blending with remaining ingredients.)

On days when I am in a rush to get out the door I will use a Tazo chai tea bag in a travel mug with the steamed milk and maple syrup, and off I go!

Ali's Sore Throat Tea

> Large mug filled with hot filtered water
> 2 drops lemon essential oil
> Juice of a fresh lemon
> Teaspoon of honey

Ali's Early Morning Detox Tea

I usually make this tea after I meditate and have my morning quiet time in my zen den downstairs. I bring it upstairs to sip as I get dressed.

> Mug of slightly warm water
> Large splash of apple cider vinegar
> Juice of half a lemon
> Teaspoon of honey

Ali's Immune Support Tea

I often make this tea from essential oils when I am sick. My dear friend Lindsay first taught me how to do this, and sometimes I vary the recipe a bit. I follow my intuition and let it guide me as to what I need. You have to be very careful when ingesting essential oils. Not all of them are meant to be ingested, so be sure you check which ones are okay! I use doTerra, which are therapeutic-grade oils.

> Hot water in a big travel mug
> Juice of a lemon

3 drops lemon oil
1 drop frankincense oil
1 drop OnGuard essential oil blend
1 drop peppermint oil
Honey to taste

Ali's "Apple Pie" Tea

Occasionally after dinner I want the taste of something sweet, but I
am full so I don't need more food. I will often enjoy a cup of "apple
pie" tea, which always satisfies my sweet tooth!

Large mug filled halfway with boiling water
Other half filled with steamed nut milk (or milk of choice)
Cinnamon apple tea bag
Honey or maple syrup to taste

Ali's Warm Weather Tea

Houston is *hot* in the summer, so I make my own version of iced tea,
but I don't always use ice! I prefer drinking things room temperature.

I fill a twenty-ounce mason jar with room temperature water
and drop in a Tulsi tea bag. Tulsi tea is caffeine-free and helps reduce
stress by maintaining cortisol levels. My favorite varieties are the
mint and lemon ginger.

If I am sitting outside in the dead of summer heat, I may throw
in some crushed ice.

Meditation #8

Nature Meditation

Let the sights and sounds of nature soothe you

In my first book *Hot Mess to Mindful Mom* I wrote about having a Trigger Plan. This is one of the first concepts that I began teaching to clients way back when. I like to say all hell can break loose in one minute, so we need to know what tools bring us back to center just as quickly! Thankfully, with this book, you'll have lots of options!

One item that is always on my trigger plan is doing a quick nature meditation. In my humble opinion, Mother Nature can help heal just about any mood, so I call on her often when I need a little pick-me-up.

I simply step outside in my backyard and breathe fresh air. I will plant my feet on the grass as I do so, and let the earth absorb and recycle any of my negative energy, and I accept an infusion of positive energy in exchange. I notice the shapes of the clouds, and I feel the air on my skin.

It's amazing how even after just one minute you feel rejuvenated and refreshed, and this can be done anywhere. Appreciate whatever elements of nature you have around you, whether you are in the city or country. If you are in a bustling city, the shapes of the clouds may become your focus. If you have more land around you, grounding your feet in the grass may be your focus. Nature is nature. Whatever piece you grab onto will work its magic.

If you live in a big city, be sure to plan weekend outings where your body can soak up the magic of Mother Earth for a more extended period of time.

And this is cool: a study was done in the Netherlands that showed that if people look at pictures with greenery (a.k.a. nature) when they were stressed, it helped bring their stress levels down. May I suggest a new screen saver?

Meditation #9

Find Something Beautiful

There is so much right in front of you

When feeling stressed or overwhelmed, another way to decrease stress is to refocus your attention on something beautiful. Try it!

Find something of beauty in your home. It can be anything, but here are a few ideas to get you started:

- A favorite piece of art
- A vase of flowers
- An empty vase that you love
- A beautiful throw pillow
- A piece of furniture that you adore

It can truly be anything that catches your eye and makes you think "that is really pretty."

Take a minute to look at it with a beginner's mind, like you've never seen it before. Appreciate it. Notice the colors and textures. Really give it your full attention.

After a minute, notice if your mind wandered at all. Did you

think about what was bothering you, or did you truly refocus your attention on that beautiful object?

Now notice how you feel. Do you feel more centered and grounded?

Meditation #10

Looking at Pictures

It's addicting!

For years I was really good about making photo albums of trips and compilations of each year. We all love to cuddle on the couch and flip through them. We laugh and share stories and remind each other of memories when one person has forgotten. We talk about which trip was our favorite, and what food we ate and can still taste in our mind.

I treasure these family times, but I also love looking at pictures of my family alone. I like to fully focus and feel all the feelings without being rushed into the next memory.

There are times I will stand in my hallway and get lost looking at pictures. Sometimes twenty or thirty minutes will go by and I have simply been staring in my boys' faces at one, two, and three years old. I silently reminisce, and I swear I can actually feel them in my arms with their head on my shoulder if I focus hard enough. I stare at those little boy cheeks and lips and get lost in the brown saucers of their eyes.

When I take the time to look at these pictures, I feel transported by love and gratitude. I feel lucky. I feel full. I relive the wonderful memories and experiences we had. I savor them quietly.

This is something we can feel anytime we look at pictures. You can transport yourself for just a minute with feelings of love. Keep a few pictures that make you feel full close by, maybe in your purse or on your desk at work. When you feel overwhelmed or anxious, take a minute to get lost in your loved ones. Put the rest of the world aside and feel all the feels.

Meditation #11

Notice Three Things

Use your surroundings

You are probably catching onto the trend in these exercises—it's all about refocusing your attention, calming down your nervous system, and coming back to center so you can move forward in your day in a more thoughtful and nourishing way. We take the opportunity to catch our breath, so to speak—maybe literally in some situations!

This exercise is great for adults and teens and can be modified slightly for younger children. It can help with anxiety, nightmares, sleep disturbances, grounding, and relaxation.

If you are doing this with a teen or child, model it for them first and then listen and stay as present as possible while they do it. If you or your child are doing this to help with sleep, and you get tired in the middle, that's good! You can stop to fall asleep.

Name three objects you see in the room, one at a time.
    Examples:
- I see the chair
- I see the light
- I see the books

- I see the door
- I see the table

Name three sounds you hear.
  Examples:
  - I hear footsteps
  - I hear the fan
  - I hear the dog
  - I hear my breath
  - I hear a car on the street

Name three feelings you are having right now.
  Examples:
  - I feel tired
  - I feel cold
  - I feel anxious
  - I feel sad
  - I feel lonely

Next: Name only two objects you see, two sounds you hear, and two things you feel.

Next: Name one object you see, one sound you hear, and one thing you feel.

This would also work really well if you need a quick break at work to refocus your energy or if a teen needs a quick study break to refocus.

Meditation #12

Power Nap

Get your timer ready!

I remember so vividly from childhood my mom's naps. She would ask me, or one of my three sisters, to wake her up in five minutes, or sometimes ten (looking back, ten must have felt luxurious).

As a typical teen, I thought this was incredibly stupid at the time! Who lies down for five minutes, and how can that even help? Well, little did I know!

My mom would immediately fall asleep, and I always felt a little guilty waking her up. This was one of many times that I learned my mom was right.

According to activebeat.com, power naps can give you that kick start of energy, especially when you take a shorter nap—the less time you nap, the less likely you'll fall into a deep sleep, which can make you groggy and take away from the potential to boost your energy.

A scientist named Rajiv Dhand outlined the effect of naps on alertness in an article titled "Good sleep, bad sleep! The role of daytime naps in healthy adults" in 2007. The study was rather extensive, but the gist was basically that a nap as short as six minutes long can improve performance and productivity, reduce fatigue, and even help you learn.

There are tips that help you get the most bang out of your power nap buck, and where else would I find them but on sleep.org? They recommend sticking to a regular napping schedule during optimal hours, which are between 1:00 p.m. and 3:00 p.m. This timeframe is optimal, since that's usually after lunchtime, when your blood sugar and energy start to dip. Do not nap for longer than thirty minutes because you run the risk of developing "sleep inertia," or that unpleasant groggy feeling that takes a considerable amount of time to shake off. And naps later than 4:00 p.m. can disrupt your regular nighttime sleep. Finally, nap in a dark room so that you'll fall asleep faster.

I get that six minutes is a touch longer than the name of this book suggests, but even though a power nap isn't exactly a one-minute meditation, it's still pretty short!

This is just one more way that I feel like my mom these days. I am starting to hear her voice in my head when I tell my kids to look at the beautiful flowers on the side of the road or notice the changing colors of the leaves on trees. Now, every time I set an alarm on my phone for a power nap, I think of her. I wonder what my kids will someday do like me that they think is weird and annoying now!

When I need a burst of energy in the afternoon, instead of reaching for caffeine that will inevitably keep me up all night, I have begun incorporating power naps into my day. I love them, just like my mom!

Meditation #13

Find Your Anchor Point

Feel the pull toward it

One of my favorite ways to start a meditation when I am guiding clients is to help them find their anchor point. We begin by relaxing the body (see Body Scan on page 77).

We then notice the sensation of the breath coming in and out of the nose. You can feel that the air feels cooler coming into your nose on the inhale and warmer as you exhale.

Next, we spend a few moments noticing the sensation of the ribcage expanding and contracting as we breathe. It's amazing how obvious this feels when you concentrate on the feeling.

Lastly, we place all our attention on the belly rising and falling as we breathe. This is called taking "belly breaths." You feel your belly expanding as you inhale and all the air leaving the belly as you exhale.

After we have done each of these three for a few minutes, I ask them to choose their anchor point. This is the place where the breath feels the strongest to them. When I am not guiding them to focus on one, which do they gravitate toward? That spot grounds them into the present moment.

This is something you can find in any moment that you need to by following the steps below:

1. Sit comfortably.
2. Close your eyes if you are in an appropriate situation to do so. If you are driving or in a meeting, or anywhere that you need to remain alert, keep your eyes open.
3. Take a breath and notice where you feel it the strongest. Is it in your nose, your ribcage, or your belly? Make this your anchor point.
4. Keep your focus on your breath in this spot for the next minute. If your mind wanders, simply return to your anchor point.

Meditation #14

Energy Check

I have learned in the past few years that I am very empathic. I soak energy up like a sponge, which can feel challenging based on where I am and who I am with.

The first time this became an issue for me was when my first book was self-published three years ago (I first self-published, then got picked up by an agent and publisher afterward). Right after its release I had a booth at a holiday bazaar to sell copies as gifts. For fourteen hours I talked to people, signed copies, and apparently soaked up a lot of energy! I spent the next five days in bed feeling like I had the flu, except I didn't. I finally reached out to my saving grace, Traci, when it finally occurred to me that I wasn't really sick; this was an energetic issue.

I learned about energy from two beautiful souls, Traci and Kayla Hines, a mother/daughter team in California. I was immediately drawn to their energy and the way that Traci, my main mentor, made the concepts around energy so relatable and easy to understand. She also taught me how to clear and protect my own energy on a daily basis so that I could stay energetically "clean," and she helped me by clearing issues that were too big for me to clear

myself. Sometimes when we are so close to a situation, we need a hand.

Traci taught me to use a pendulum to help keep my analytical mind from overriding my ability to connect with energy that needed to be cleared from other people, as well as my own energy fields. The pendulum lets me know when each stage of clearing is complete and helps me tap into my intuitive awareness without getting stuck in the chatter of my mind.

My journey over the past few years with this has been extraordinary. I have grown so much, and I've gained skills that help make my day-to-day life so much more peaceful. Traci and I still talk about once a month to this day, because I am always growing and reaching new stages of awareness and development. As I become more visible in the world I have her on my team to help me clear bigger issues. It is so interesting to discuss them with her, and we always have major celebrations because I am able to now tap into where the energy is coming from in many cases, or catch it myself and clear it, without sending her constant SOS texts. It feels very empowering to understand these concepts.

It is important to mention that 99.9 percent of people are not sending you negative energy on purpose. It is usually totally subconscious, and they have no clue. Here's an example of how this can happen: Let's say you post a beautiful sunset picture from an amazing vacation in Hawaii and someone sees it as they sit on their couch during a snowstorm. They are thinking about how they want to go on vacation, and they haven't had a proper vacation in so long. As they stew in feeling sorry for themselves some of that energy is sent to you without their ever realizing it.

I love the way the Universe works, and now I have people reaching out to me to do an energetic clearing for them or to teach them how to do them. This wasn't my intention when I began learning,

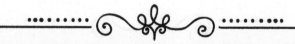

but I trust the guidance I receive, and when three people in one week asked me to do clearings for them, I took it as a sign that this would now be part of what I can offer the world.

I get so excited and actually feel many physical sensations as I am performing clearings for people, usually based on what energy is being released. It is very cool. I am now clearing the energy that a client picks up from other people and situations, as well as their energy fields relating to things like forgiveness, inherited traits, authenticity, trust, fear, life purpose, relationships, and more. I love when I communicate to a sitter (the person I'm doing the clearing for) what I am feeling and they say, "Well, that makes sense!"

I begin each day by protecting my energy for the day and end every day by clearing it. I take a few minutes and run through various steps and questions, and it's now part of my routine. I also take little breaks throughout the day to clear and protect based on the people I interact with and the situations I'm in. It isn't always convenient to whip out my pendulum (especially when driving!), even though I never leave home without one, but intention works just as well, and that's what I want you to take away from this.

A mid-day clear or protect can be a one-minute meditation. Call on whomever/whatever feels comfortable to you—some like Higher Self, Universe, Archangel Michael—it will all work because your intention is what matters! You can stop whatever you are doing, close your eyes, and with intention (this is the important part!) say something to the effect of:

"Please protect my energy now. Please put a golden bubble of light around me that nothing may penetrate except love, light, and pure connection. Please let anything not meant for me and my highest good bounce off this bubble and return to its sender."

Now picture yourself being surrounded in a golden bubble of light that will be your energetic armor.

Some good times to use protection would be:

- As the phone rings and you see a name that always throws you into a tizzy.
- Before you walk into a meeting that your intuition tells you may feel a bit hostile.
- Before you are going to a public or crowded space if you feel sensitive to a lot of energy.
- Every morning!

If you feel that you have picked up energy that doesn't belong to you, you can do pretty much the same thing by saying something like this, and addressing it to Higher Self, the Universe, Archangel Michael, or whatever you're comfortable with:

"Please clear any energy that I may have picked up that doesn't belong to me. Please hit return to sender and give it back to the original owner. Please send it back with love and light, and detach my energy completely."

Some good times to use this prayer would be:

- After a phone call that didn't feel good or with a very negative person.
- If you feel your energy dipping during the day. Maybe you picked something up that isn't yours.
- Anytime you leave a crowded or public place.
- Every night!

These prayers take less than a minute, but can change the course of your entire day. You don't have to wait until bedtime to check in with your energy.

Meditation #15

On Location

Your phone is a mindfulness tool

If I told you there was something you could do in about ten seconds to boost your mood, increase feelings of positivity, help attract what you want, and raise your vibration all at the same time, would you do it? I would!

Welcome to the world of affirmations.

What exactly are they? The actual definition succinctly states that using affirmations is the practice of positive thinking and self-empowerment—fostering a belief that "a positive mental attitude supported by affirmations will achieve success in anything." More specifically, an affirmation is a carefully formatted statement that should be repeated to one self and written down frequently. For affirmations to be effective, it is said that they need to be present tense, positive, personal, and specific.

I use affirmations all the time, but to be completely honest I haven't done that much research on them—I was simply drawn to the practice because it felt good. Affirmations 100 percent make me refocus my attention to something positive and uplifting. So, when I wanted to find out more, I of course turned to the work of Louise Hay, the queen of affirmations.

The benefits of affirmations:

Louise died in 2017, but her work lives on. She was an inspirational teacher who educated millions since the 1984 publication of her bestseller, *You Can Heal Your Life*, about the healing power of affirmations.

Louise has written a lot about affirmations, so I will let you hear it right from her. She states:

> An affirmation opens the door. It's a beginning point on the path to change. In essence, you're saying to your subconscious mind: *"I am taking responsibility. I am aware that there is something I can do to change."* When I talk about *doing affirmations,* I mean consciously choosing words that will either help *eliminate* something from your life or help *create* something new in your life.
>
> Every thought you think and every word you speak is an affirmation. All of our self-talk, our internal dialogue, is a stream of affirmations. You're using affirmations every moment whether you know it or not. You're affirming and creating your life experiences with every word and thought.
>
> Your beliefs are merely habitual thinking patterns that you learned as a child. Many of them work very well for you. Other beliefs may be limiting your ability to create the very things you say you want. What you want and what you believe you deserve may be very different. You need to pay attention to your thoughts so that you can begin to eliminate the ones creating experiences you do *not* want in your life.
>
> Please realize that every complaint is an affirmation of something you don't want in your life. Every time you get

angry, you're affirming that you want more anger in your life. Every time you feel like a victim, you're affirming that you want to *continue* to feel like a victim. If you feel that life isn't giving you what you want in your world, then it's certain that you will never have the goodies that life gives to others—that is, until you change the way you think and talk.

You're not a bad person for thinking the way you do. You've just never learned *how* to think and talk. People throughout the world are just now beginning to learn that our thoughts create our experiences. Your parents probably didn't know this, so they couldn't possibly teach it to you. They taught you how to look at life in the way that *their* parents taught them. So nobody is wrong. However, it's time for all of us to wake up and begin to consciously create our lives in a way that pleases and supports us. *You* can do it. *I* can do it. *We all* can do it—we just need to learn how.

So. So. Good.

She makes such an important point about how our negative self-talk is like an affirmation for what we don't want. I don't think many people think about it like that, but we all should! This is why affirmations need to be positive and present tense.

I have a very favorite affirmation that I use almost daily when I am feeling stressed or overwhelmed. I state, "I get everything done with ease and grace." It immediately calms me when my to-do list feels insurmountable, and it helps me stay centered and grounded in positive feelings.

Even though I love public speaking, and I traveled to seven different states this past year to do it, I still get nervous right before.

It's like I am so excited to give the speech, then for the five minutes before it starts I want to throw up and I ask myself why I can't just be a quiet girl, and then right when my mouth opens I am in my zone and afterward I feel on top of the world. Every time! But who wants to feel like they are going to throw up before something exciting? I started using an affirmation to help and I say, "You were born for this." It raises my vibration and puts me in a state of mind to shine on that stage. Even though "were" is technically past tense, "this" is present and the part that matters. I am sticking with it because it always works!

A hack to remember to use them:

The only problem with affirmations is that it can be hard to remember to use them. As good as our intentions are, life is busy, so reminders are definitely helpful. I am big on reminders because I need them to stay on track with my practices.

I have found that sticky notes are good, but in the age of technology, my smartphone is actually a great mindfulness tool when it comes to affirmations. I programed affirmations into my reminder feature so that an affirmation flashes on my screen hourly, and when I see it I take a deep breath and repeat it a few times, like a one-minute meditation.

Here is a sampling of the ones I use:

- I am here to serve. I always serve to the best of my ability.
- I am supported by the Universe. My books are supported by the Universe.
- My intention for today is _____(I fill it in each day).
- It's this or something better. Everything happens in divine timing.

- I speak my truth always, in all ways.
- Joy in everything I do.
- Gratitude is my attitude.
- I am connected, protected, guided, and directed. (This one came from Rebecca Rosen. If you don't know who she is you have to read my first book, *Hot Mess to Mindful Mom*!)

But here's the coolest part. On an iPhone (Android peeps, you may have a way to set this as well!) you can have a reminder/affirmation flash at a particular location. Think about it—you can pull into carpool line and an affirmation can pop up that says, "I am a present and centered mommy." You can pull into work and it could flash, "I am confident in all my decisions at work." The possibilities are endless.

Take a moment and think about your day. Where would affirmations help you the most? Write one for that particular situation and program the location for where you want it to flash across your screen. So cool!

Meditation #16

Take One Thing Away

Sometimes one thing has just gotta go

I aim to be very respectful of my calendar and treat it like a friend, but occasionally it gets away from me. Every once in a while it makes me break out into a cold sweat. These are the times when I need to get a grip and use one of these tools that I am sharing with you!

When I feel my heart palpitating, I know something has to go.

Over the years I have come to rely on my body's wisdom. Sometimes my brain gets confused, but my gut always knows what's up! My body speaks to me (the cold sweats and heart palpitations!), and so does yours. Please, I'm begging you, don't ignore its signals.

After a lot of practice, I have gained lots of awareness of how to help myself best in these circumstances of overwhelm.

First thing: *Stop.*

Second thing: **Breathe**—a few deep breaths to immediately chill.

Third thing: Focus my breathing, usually a one-minute meditation of inhale for three and exhale for three.

Fourth thing: Do a quick body scan if I need it to calm myself down even more.

Fifth thing: Evaluate my calendar and *take one thing away*.

Sixth thing: Use the affirmation "I get everything done with ease and grace" for everything that is left because it can still be busy!

There is one thing I have learned for sure over the years, and that is that I can't do it all. I can't be everything to everyone, and I can't fill every single time slot on my calendar and be good to anyone, especially myself. I turn into a stressed-out mess!

In my early days of teaching I had been known to get a little overzealous and overcommit. My family will be the first to tell you it happened. It makes me a tiny bit sad to even admit it, but it came from a place of passion and excitement. I said yes to everything. I was so excited to spread the message about the incredible benefits of meditation and mindfulness, and I felt like it was the beginning of people truly getting it and wanting to know more about it.

My family always jokes that I have incredible timing! I left Enron six months before the collapse, and I began teaching meditation right before you started hearing about it and reading about it everywhere. That is my hope with now also teaching Kundalini Yoga. I think people are ready for it, and my timing is great!

So I was saying yes to every volunteer opportunity and paying client. Three nights in a row, how could I say no?

But in all honesty, I was spending a few too many nights away from my family, missing tuck-ins and snuggles. I didn't work for myself to miss out on my family; it was supposed to be the opposite.

Every newbie and entrepreneur has to pay their dues to a certain extent and put in the time and effort to make their business a success. It was easy to do this because I wanted to serve and share. I loved it so much. But I loved my family more, so I could see that I needed some ground rules.

Ground rules:

1. When my calendar sends me into a panic, I have to remove one thing from it, or reschedule to another date.
2. I only teach one night a week. I will not miss more tuck-ins than that.
3. Work travel for speaking will be as quick as possible, approximately twenty-four hours including travel, so I only miss one tuck-in.
4. I will say yes to one volunteer opportunity a month. I can't say yes to everyone at the same time.

You can see that tuck-ins are my priority right now. My boys won't want me to tuck them in forever, so I don't want to miss too many of those snuggles and wonderful conversations that happen before bed.

Things don't usually get removed from the calendar altogether; they simply get moved to a day with more breathing room. Sometimes it has to be coffee or lunch with a friend if I have too many work commitments that just can't be moved. I have had to cancel on my trainer and take a walk before dinner instead. I never reschedule clients, but sometimes there is flexibility on meeting times or phone calls. I do a lot of connecting with other entrepreneurs, and thankfully they get it too!

Be honest with yourself. Do you completely thrive on a full calendar, or do you go into a panic like me? If so, be mindful of how you enter things. Are you giving yourself breathing room and time to transition? If not, think about what ground rules you need and put them into action.

Meditation #17

Stretch Those Muscles

Your body will thank you!

I have many strengths in my life but flexibility is not one of them! I have worked on it on and off throughout my adult life, and have gotten more serious since I started practicing more Kundalini Yoga.

One of the problems is that I will stretch well one day, then run the next, and forget to stretch! So I tighten right back up.

What I have learned is that stretching is no different than any other self-care tool—it's about consistency and using the tools. Like I always say, "tools only work if you work them." This goes for me just like all of my clients!

It's all about sneaking some of your tools into your life so they feel seamless and just part of your everyday routine. I was looking for a way to get more stretching in, so I decided to do it in the shower.

I came up with this because I started using a new line of shampoo. You are supposed to do two washes and conditioner, and each one is one to two minutes. Some of that time is obviously taken up with washing with soap, and maybe shaving, but I had some extra time on my hands!

I started doing one-minute meditations, saying prayers, and stretching. It was a really good use of my time!

The more I stretch, the more I want to because it feels good and mentally I know I am working toward a goal of touching toes. Even if you are more flexible, stretching is still important to maintain flexibility and range of motion.

In times of stress and overwhelm, stretching is another great option for a one-minute meditation. It's a wonderful way to re-focus your attention and get grounded in your body. Stretching can be done in your living room or a bathroom stall. All you need is yourself!

Meditation #18

Music to Recalibrate

Get ready to jam!

Some things are just intuitive. You do them without thinking about them. Like picking a song to listen to that fits your current mood.

When I am happy, I want to jam. I dance in my car, and I've even been known to stop on the sidewalk when a really fun song comes on during a run and have a one-person dance party right there on the street. I couldn't care less what anyone thinks. I am in the moment!

When I want to feel really connected to my soul, I pull up my "meditation playlist" full of Sanskrit and Gurmukhi lyrics and it always makes me feel grounded and centered to chant the words. I love to chant while I am cooking or driving, and even though my kids complain when I play them in the car, they know all the words and totally sing along! I do use music when I practice Kundalini Yoga, which makes the practice even more amazing than it already is because I love the music so much.

I have also found that a song can change my mood, and a one- or two-minute dance party can completely recalibrate my energy, so even though it isn't anything quiet or seated, I often use a quick song

and dance break to bust through blocks or shift my feelings when I need to. I sing to my dogs at the top of my lungs and what I do is probably considered more jumping around than awesome dancing, but it feels great!

One of the really fun parts of writing a book is researching topics that you have only thought about at more of a surface level. I know music affects me and changes my mood, but I've never really looked into it, so to speak.

For example, have you ever wondered exactly why we want to hear sad songs after a breakup? A study published in the Journal of Consumer Research suggested that sad music provides a substitute for the lost relationship. They compared it to the preference most people have for an empathic friend—someone who truly understands what you're going through. I've never thought of it that way before!

Other research has focused on the joy upbeat music can bring. A 2013 study in the Journal of Positive Psychology found that people who listened to upbeat music could improve their moods and boost their happiness in just two weeks. So maybe I need to make my singalong dance breaks a daily occurrence.

I do like country, but I am really a chart pop fan at heart. I love the Top 40 countdowns, and I could really bond with a twelve-year-old over music! My nieces and I could totally swap playlists.

The Top 40 charts are easy to come by, but I thought it would be fun to share some of my favorite music for chanting, contemplation, and grounding. This may be new to you so keep an open mind and give them a try! I find them so beautiful.

- "Gobinday Mukunday" by Snatam Kaur
- "Ong Namo" by Ajeet Kaur

- "Gobinday" by Mukunday by Gurunam Singh
- "Sa Ta Na Ma" by Mantra Girl
- "Guru Ram Das Chant" by Snatam Kaur
- "Beautiful, Blissful" by Harnam
- "Long Time Sun" by Snatam Kuar
- "I Am Light" by India Arie
- "Aad Guray Nameh" by Jai-Jagdeesh
- "Love, Serve & Remember" by John Astin
- "Sa Re Sa Sa" by Nirinjan Kaur
- "Baba Hanuman" by Shantala
- "Sat Siri Siri Akal" by Shunia

I hope you enjoy them as much as I do!

Next time you are feeling sad, overwhelmed, or just *blah* for whatever reason, use your intuition to pick a song that will help you change that. One day it may be something uplifting and fun, and another it may be a chant to ground you. Play with it and see what you are drawn to.

Meditation #19

Breathing Square

For the visual learners

There are so many things I love about meditation—there is something for everyone! You may gravitate to a few of these tools and want to stick with them, or you may incorporate different ones into your routine all the time. The best news: there is no right or wrong way to do it!

This goes for a longer seated meditation or a quick one-minute meditation. Some people like to pick one breathing exercise or mantra and stick with it, and others like variety. I personally fall into the second category.

Whether I am doing a longer seated meditation when I wake up in the morning or a quickie sometime throughout the day, I always check in with my body and ask it what it needs. Sometimes a mantra pops into my head, sometimes a certain way to breathe, sometimes an affirmation, and other times a body scan. I use all of the tools in this book at different times based on what I need in the moment. I have found that I gravitate toward some more than others, but they are all in rotation.

You can decide to do the same thing. Check in with yourself, or if that feels too complicated, or you tend to be indecisive, then choose one or two go-to's and stick with them.

Another option is to test out both ways and see what works. I am a very decisive person. I pick something and go with it, whether it is bathroom tile, a pair of jeans, or a one-minute meditation. I don't waver and I don't look back. It's forward motion for me! My older son, on the other hand, is the opposite, so he would spend five minutes picking what to do in his one-minute meditation. He's much better off with one or two choices. You have to figure out what works for you!

I really love using a breathing square for a few reasons. It helps to reduce stress and anxiety, as well as lower cortisol hormones and calm the nervous system, just like all of these quick exercises.

One aspect that sets this one apart is that it can be great for auditory, visual, and kinesthetic learners alike.

Approximately 65 percent of the population are visual learners, 30 percent are auditory, and 5 percent are tactile learners, with again, most people being a combination of these learner styles. It's important as a teacher to find ways to accommodate all kind of learners, and the breathing square is a great option. It is also wonderful for kids as well as adults for just this reason.

Using the breathing square is pretty simple. The breath counts are as follows:

1. Inhale for a count of four.
2. Hold your breath in for a count of four.
3. Exhale for a count of four.
4. Hold the exhale out for a count of four.
5. Repeat.

For auditory learners I can simply give these instructions and let them proceed because that is really all they need.

For more tactile learners, I may have them close their eyes and draw a square on their thigh as they breathe, so they can feel the square being made on their body.

For visual learners, I will use this picture of a breathing square and have them move their fingers along the lines with their eyes open so they can watch the square being made.

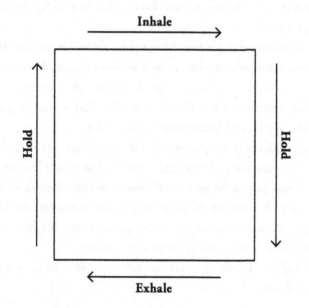

If the visual is helpful, you can draw a square on any scrap piece of paper and follow along with your finger. Drawing on your thigh can also be done in a pinch with eyes open or closed to accommodate more visual and tactile learners. I consider this a catch-all meditation that really appeals to everyone since there are so many ways to use it. Kids especially love it, so definitely teach yours!

Meditation #20

Feel Your Feelings

Denial won't get you anywhere

Sometimes I feel like a broken record. My clients have heard this multiple times:

"Every feeling is okay, but not every reaction to every feeling is okay!"

Oh, and this one:

"We can't get around feelings, we can only go through them."

But you know what? They don't get sick of hearing them because they are true, and we always need little reminders to stay on track.

When we ignore our feelings they can potentially create emotional blocks for us, which can lead to dis-ease in the body, and trust me, the same situation will continue to present itself in your life until you finally change your thought patterns and the way you react to it.

Pushing feelings aside, or ignoring them until you are alone, can understandably feel like self-preservation in the moment. It may not be the right time or place to deal with an emotion, and that's okay. That's why it's important to become aware of what thoughts and feelings need to be dealt with, and make the effort to come back to them at a more appropriate time to give them the attention they deserve.

When you have a moment to focus on you, and whatever thought or feeling needs to be processed, set the intention to truly feel it and move through it.

Sit with your eyes closed in a safe, comfortable place, preferably alone.

Think about whatever emotion, situation, or thought you want to focus on. You can do this as many times as you need to for different things.

When you bring up the thought, emotion, or memory, where do you feel it in your body?

What does it feel like? Does it have a color? Is it big or small?

Stay with the feeling and notice if it moves. Notice if it lessens or intensifies.

Give it your undivided attention.

Send it feelings of love, almost like a little baby that needs to be rocked and comforted.

Keep paying attention until it lessens or disappears.

Repeat as needed for the same emotion, thought, or memory until you feel neutral about it in your body.

Feeling your feelings in this way allows you to give them the attention they deserve instead of brushing them aside, and possibly ignoring them forever, which will only lead to problems later.

Meditation #21

Wave Your Magic Wand

A realistic one

The story of how I got into coaching is as "whoo-whoo" as how I got into meditation (that is the best story ever, in my first book *Hot Mess to Mindful Mom*!), but I love that stuff so I'm always happy to share my awesomely out-there experiences!

I had been teaching meditation for almost a year, when I was sitting in a deep meditation myself. I remember so distinctly sitting cross-legged in a leather chair in a hotel room in San Antonio, with earbuds in as my family watched television early in the morning. An unmistakable voice popped into my head, sounding very male, just like the voice I wrote about in the introduction, and it said out of the clear blue, "Coaching is the next step for you."

I had never thought about my next steps. I didn't even know there were next steps yet! I was so happy teaching meditation and I hadn't thought beyond it, but I took this guidance seriously because I always trust messages I receive and am grateful that the Universe is giving me clues, almost like breadcrumbs to follow down my life path.

That next week I was dropping my son off at a playdate, and the mom, who is a friend of mine, asked me how work was going. I said great, and threw out there that I was now going to be coaching. It was the first time I even said it out loud . . . and she hired me on the spot. What a wink from the Universe. In that moment it was truly a confirmation that this was indeed my next step.

I loved coaching from that very first client. So many of my clients were moms, and they all wanted to talk about issues with their kids, so I began coaching around self-care and mindful parenting. I felt confident from the get-go, and it all felt very intuitive, but I decided to gain additional skills to become the best coach I could be.

I began learning from Christian Mickelsen and Susan Epstein, two renowned coaches in the areas of general life coaching and parenting coaching. I acquired new skills which I put into action right away, and my clients saw empowering results.

It was so fulfilling to work with people for longer periods of time, and help them see major success and their goals being achieved. This led me to also change the structure of my meditation business a bit.

When I first started teaching, I said "yes" to every opportunity. I was building a business and I was too scared to say "no" to anything. If someone wanted one session, fine. I just wanted to build a client base in any way possible and get as much teaching experience as I could. I learned a few things from this:

- I am a *very* good teacher. I have the ability to make the huge, sometimes intimidating concepts of meditation and mindfulness feel relatable and accessible.
- I want to see my clients succeed, and they couldn't with a one-and-done lesson.
- I wanted longer-term commitments from my meditation students so that they could reach their goals of having a solid

meditation practice at home. I would only teach people willing to come to me at least three times to start. After that I could be more flexible if they wanted pop-ins to stay on track.

- My new standards meant I wasn't the right teacher for everyone out there, and that's okay!
- I was willing to see fewer students, because my terms were very important to me. I knew in my heart and gut this was best to help people succeed.

I also found that I liked the variety of teaching meditation and coaching each week. Doing both kept me invigorated, and I was constantly using my entire skill set, which always challenged me.

When I speak to a potential new coaching client, my job is to ask the right questions and then shut up and listen. The potential client does most of the talking during those intro sessions. Thanks to my training, I know what questions to ask to get them to really open up, and they end up sharing things that they didn't even realize they needed and wanted to work on.

My very favorite question is the Magic Wand. I ask them, "If you had a real magic wand, what would your life look like?" They then tell me what their ideal life would look like in terms of work and personal life, friendships, travel, habits, and what it would feel like inside. Then I ask them, "What is standing in your way of having that?" and that is where the real investigation begins, and what they share is the beginning stages of the work they need to do. I give them opportunity after opportunity to dig deeper and to surprise themselves with what they find when they don't stop looking right away.

These calls are usually a full hour, and are pretty all-encompassing in terms of what we cover, but there are ways to break this question down for yourself in times of struggle, almost like a one-minute meditation.

Instead of looking at your entire life at once, if you are struggling in a particular situation, or in moving forward with a conversation, or in dealing with a feeling or emotion, use these questions:

- If I waved a real magic wand, what would this one situation look like, or feel like? How would I handle this conversation?
- What's standing in my way?

The awareness that can come from taking the moment necessary to ask yourself these questions before moving forward in a way you may regret is life altering. Nothing can change without first having awareness, so congratulate yourself on the miracle of noticing and asking. By asking these questions you are claiming your desire to know yourself on a deeper level. You are getting to the heart of the matter, instead of just floating along listlessly. You have the power to change your life by asking these important questions.

Meditation #22

Self-Love

Life. Changing.

I have been on a self-love journey for the past seven years. It started by default, honestly not realizing it at all. I wasn't aware that I needed more self-love, mostly because it was the "hot mess" phase of my life and I didn't know that things could feel different. I was focused on the wrong things, what everyone was doing, instead of what was going on inside of me at a body, mind, and soul level.

I didn't have a moment where I stated "I need to practice more self-love" like a proclamation or anything of the sort, but my habits began to change. I incorporated more self-care, which in turn created a more loving and nurturing environment for my soul, and a whole lot more self-awareness. It was a process, and just like anything worthwhile in life, it took time and commitment.

Even though I didn't set out to begin a self-love journey, the more I meditated and practiced mindfulness and self-care, the better I felt, so the more I wanted to do.

Peeling back the onion

It's interesting, as different situations and experiences surface, they peel back more layers, kind of like an onion, and highlight what we still need to heal in our lives.

Writing this book actually catapulted me into a new phase of self-love and acceptance as wounds that needed to be healed showed themselves.

I was baffled because my first two books, *Hot Mess to Mindful Mom* and *Get the Most out of Motherhood* literally flew out of me. I wrote them with ease as the words spilled out every single day until they were completed. The process felt fun and breezy. Then there was this book, which felt like I did a 180-degree turn.

I made every excuse not to write, both legitimate and not, for months. We took a huge family trip to Israel in honor of my son's and niece's B'nai Mitzvah which required a ton of planning, and then we also had a celebration in Houston a few months later. If you have never planned a Bar Mitzvah it can feel like planning a wedding. It was the most joyous and special occasion, but it took uber amounts of time. I began to feel so stressed and pulled with writing at the same time that I decided to simply shut my computer off for two months and focus on my son and this milestone. I wanted to enjoy it to the max, and it definitely felt like the right choice. Those were the legitimate excuses.

After the exhaustion subsided it was time to jump back into writing with both feet, but I was still dragging. I actually had one, only one, moment where I contemplated returning my advance and just saying "no" to this process. But something stopped me. I looked at my outline and I was so compelled and enthusiastic about the material that I was writing. I wanted these tools to get out into the world in an accessible way for more people to handle stress in the moment and better their lives. I loved my outline and I couldn't stop. I wanted to bring this book to the world. I had to figure out a way to move through my writing drought and whatever blocks were stopping me.

When you are brave enough to ask for answers, the Universe will usually provide them. In the midst of writing a book and celebrating the Bar Mitzvah, I had started Kundalini Yoga teacher training (more on that in a bit). I was deep in meditation one morning of training and feelings began to surface that proved to be life-altering. I became aware of wounds around self-worth and self-love that I needed to pay attention to. The most simple way to explain it is that this book became a symbol of the need to prove that I still felt deep within.

I saw the big picture of my life and career in a new light, and it became obvious that growing up with lack created a drive in me to constantly prove my worth by constantly doing more. I felt this deep-seated need to show that I was just as deserving as everyone else when it came to success and a happy and fulfilled life.

Writing one book wasn't good enough to prove this. Writing two books didn't fill the void. So, maybe a third would?

I finally understood that no amount of books could fill this hole. No amount of speaking engagements, or clients, or likes on Instagram or Facebook. This was the tough stuff. This was about the internal work and unconditional self-love and self-worth that I needed to continue to cultivate.

I had to do enough soul-searching to understand that if I never give one more speech or write another word, I am still enough. I am good enough. I am deserving of my dreams. I am deserving of the wonderful life Mark and I have built together. I don't have anything to prove. I am enough just as I am.

Admitting that I still had work to do around this opened me up in new ways, and I spent a few weeks really contemplating these issues and feelings. For a few weeks this process consumed

my thoughts, my journal, and my walks and runs. I spoke to a few trusted souls about it, including my Kundalini Yoga teacher trainer. She told me that the fact that I became aware of these wounds and feelings is a miracle. Most people go through life never understanding where the blocks come from.

This book turned out to be the catalyst for deep soul healing. It was the way the Universe got my attention that something was up. I literally felt like a new person as soon as I began to bring these feelings from so deep inside of me to the surface. It was freeing.

And you know what? After they came up, the book started flowing, and I was once again writing from my heart with ease. It was a relief like no other, especially as my deadline was approaching!

I had always heard that Kundalini Yoga teacher training could bring up some deep things, and boy, were my friends correct! There was more around self-love that needed to be healed.

After that deep meditation something else happened as well. All of my classmates went to lunch and I had a strong feeling that I needed to be alone. I ended up sitting outside on the front porch of the ashram, bawling. A more accurate description may be wailing with a slow transition to a flow of tears that needed to pour out for a very long time. Overwhelming sadness came over me, but it felt like such a release at the same time. In my morning meditation I saw scenes of my life pass before my eyes. They were all of the hardest situations and experiences I've had from growing up, but interestingly I met them with neutrality. It was like a movie playing for me. Since I'd done so much work in the past few years around forgiveness, they no longer affected me in the same way, but on that porch I began to cry for the little girl that endured those experiences. I was so sad for her and my tears were the release I needed to process these feelings. I told her I was so, so sorry that she had to endure hardship

and sadness, and feel so insecure. I told her that it wasn't fair, and I wish it were different for her. I assured that scared little girl that I loved her, and that she was now safe. This was one of the most healing acts I have ever taken part in.

What is self-love?

So, what is self-love exactly, and how do we practice more of it? I think everyone's definition is personal. I can share with you what mine is. There are six key principles that have helped me construct a healthier relationship with myself, and they are as follows.

Accepting myself: I have come to truly accept myself, including all of my challenges and gifts. Using mindfulness, which is moment-to-moment awareness without judgment, means that I understand, accept, and embrace that everything won't be perfect all of the time, including me.

Having boundaries: I have learned to have better boundaries with myself and others. I say "yes" when my heart is truly in something, and I politely decline when it's not. I realize that I can't be everything to everyone, and that sometimes I may disappoint someone else to be true to myself.

Forgiving myself: As hard as I try to do the right things, say the right things, and plan well, I will make mistakes. I will occasionally say and do things that I regret, and the only thing I can do is apologize from my heart and be more careful in the future by mindfully slowing down, choosing words and actions thoughtfully.

There is nothing good that will come from rehashing mistakes in my mind for days, months, or years. I will learn whatever lesson

can be extracted from the situation or experience and move forward with the knowledge and understanding of what I would do differently next time.

Intentional living: I love myself enough to fill my days with nourishing behaviors such as meditation, exercise, healthy eating, time in nature, and loving relationships. These are priorities in my life and are part of my self-care plan.

If a person or activity causes me undue stress, I will do my best to limit my exposure and prioritize clearing and protecting my energy at that time.

Listening to my intuition: It is said that we have three brains—our gut, our heart, and the one in our head. Our intuition usually speaks to us through our gut feelings and instincts, and trusting these intuitive hits is part of practicing self-love. I have learned to love myself enough to listen. More on this later.

Believing I am worthy: This is the key—you must believe you are worthy of your own love.

Self-love rituals

Self-love rituals help me daily to acknowledge how important I am in my own life, and how deserving of my own love I am.

I use this practice at the end of each of my daily meditations because it feels so good. I place my hands on my heart center and I say out loud, *"I love you, Ali. I love you. I am proud of you. You are enough. You do enough. I love you."*

It feels so good I find myself smiling each time I do it. I truly feel it, and I know it may sound silly, but you just have to try it. I even have teens do it when they learn from me, and they love it! You can also think it in your head and say it silently, but I think it is much more powerful if you say it aloud.

I also use this tool as a one-minute meditation, and I find I gravitate toward it after I have made a mistake. I can occasionally berate myself for saying something really stupid. I'll think about it and feel embarrassed all over again every few minutes. This isn't productive or very mindful behavior, and even though it doesn't happen as much as it used to, thank goodness, occasionally I fall back into this pattern. I'm human, after all!

When I find myself in this negative spiral I use a tool as quickly as I can to pull myself back to reality and the present moment, and this self-love affirmation, spoken with my hands on my heart with clear intention, always seems to make me feel better. *I love you, Ali. I forgive you. You are human. It's okay. I love you. I love you.*

See how good it feels after your meditations, and any time you need a little boost or pick me up. It's one of my favorites!

Meditation #23

I Am . . .

What Follows Can Change Your Trajectory

Houston lived through Hurricane Harvey in 2017, and our neighborhood was hit especially hard. We had so many friends that were displaced and had to completely redo their homes. It became truly obvious why it's called a natural disaster. People's lives were turned upside down, not to mention the feelings of helplessness and loss that everyone in the city felt.

In comparison to what many friends and loved ones were going through, we were extremely lucky. Our garage flooded, and we sustained damage outside of our home, but the interior living space was spared. We threw ourselves into helping others in need to salvage and pack what they could, and I felt useful feeding friends and loved ones, so I had people over for meals as much as possible. It's the Jewish mother in me!

I'd say the only silver lining to Harvey is seeing the way that the Houston community pulled together in such a trying time. Everyone did what they could to help loved ones and strangers alike. My sons' school flooded very badly, and families turned out in

droves to help pull up carpets, scrape glue off tile floors, knock out walls that needed to be replaced, and anything else to help get our kids back in school. We had some major motivation!

Another complete devastation to our community was that our synagogue flooded, and the entire sanctuary was ruined. We are the largest conservative temple in the country. Four thousand families celebrate milestones and worship there, and the question on everyone's mind was "Where will High Holidays services be held?" Harvey happened a few weeks before Rosh Hashanah and Yom Kippur, which are the Jewish New Year and Day of Atonement, respectively.

Day in and day out I drive by Lakewood Church. Joel Osteen is the pastor there, and most people have heard of him. I have occasionally turned on the television in foreign countries, and no matter what language is spoken there, Joel Osteen is on the screen Sunday mornings with his sermons being translated. Lakewood Church is so big that their facility used to be where the Houston Rockets played. It is literally as big as a stadium, and it gets filled to the brim every weekend. I had a gut feeling that our displaced Jewish community just may end up there for our holiday services. It was the only place that seemed big enough to hold us!

In a compassionate display of humanity, the Osteens did indeed open their church to our synagogue for High Holiday services. I have to say, I felt welcomed in a way that touched my heart completely. The church volunteers were warm and friendly, and offered the traditional Hebrew New Year greeting, *L'Shana Tova*. We were made to feel right at home. It was lovely.

I left services with a soft spot for Joel Osteen and Lakewood Church, which makes it even more special to share his explanation about words that are very meaningful to me. In the following passage, Osteen explains why what words follow "I am" are so vitally important:

Here's the principle. *Whatever follows the "I am" will eventually find you.* When you say, "I am so clumsy," clumsiness comes looking for you. "I am so old." Wrinkles come looking for you. "I am so overweight." Calories come looking for you. It's as though you're inviting them. Whatever you follow the "I am" with, you're handing it an invitation, opening the door, and giving it permission to be in your life. The good news is you get to choose what follows the "I am."

When you go through the day saying, "I am blessed," blessings come looking for you. "I am talented." Talent comes looking for you. You may not feel up to par, but when you say, "I am healthy," health starts heading your way. "I am strong." Strength starts tracking you down. You're inviting those things into your life. That's why you have to be careful what follows the "I am." Don't ever say, "I am so unlucky. I never get any good breaks." You're inviting disappointments. "I am so broke. I am so in debt." You are inviting struggle. You're inviting lack.

You need to send out some new invitations. Get up in the morning and invite good things into your life. "I am blessed. I am strong. I am talented. I am wise. I am disciplined. I am focused. I am prosperous." When you talk like that, talent gets summoned by Almighty God: "Go find that person." Health, strength, abundance, and discipline start heading your way.

I believe strongly in the power of our words. I talk about

conscious language all the time, to the point of pausing and correcting myself in the moment if I say something which doesn't resonate with how I truly feel inside, or how I want to feel. If I use language inviting what I *don't want* into my life by accident, I turn it around right then and there. I'm not embarrassed to say, "wait . . . that's not how I want to put that. Let me take a do-over right now."

One of my favorite phrases to use is "I am peace." When I feel overwhelmed or frustrated I will repeat this silently to myself for a minute and I feel myself calm, and truly feel peaceful inside. Then I can carry on with whatever I need to do, feeling much more in control of my emotions because I am connected to the peaceful center within.

Here are a few more phrases that feel wonderful with "I am" and will invite positive feelings into your day:

- I am loved.
- I am a calm and loving parent.
- I am destined for great things.
- I am an excellent public speaker.
- I am appreciated by my loved ones.
- I am a good friend.
- I am healthy and strong.
- I am happy.
- I am abundant.
- I am beautiful.
- I am creative.
- I am capable.
- I am centered.
- I am forgiving.

- I am grateful.
- I am strength.
- I am worthy of . . .

Give one minute to an "I am" affirmation and see how you feel after a few days. You can use a different one every day, or use the same one for a week or two.

You can make an "I am" statement your screen saver, or post a note on your fridge to see throughout the day to take this practice to the next level.

Meditation #24

Mindful Eating

One bite at a time

I am a dark chocolate-aholic. One hundred percent. I don't eat tons of sweets, but I have a square of seventy percent or higher every day after lunch and dinner. It is part of my routine, and I don't care if it is solid dark, almond sea salt, mint, or any other variety. I usually mix it up when buying my weekly bars.

Most days I gobble that square in one or two bites, walking through my kitchen, or adding something to my calendar. However, occasionally I make this sweet treat an event.

I stop whatever I am doing and I actually sit down, usually on the stool at my kitchen island, which is my favorite place to sit if I am alone. In fact, I don't think I have sat down alone to eat at an actual table in years! The sitting signifies that this is a major mindful moment.

I take a moment to look at the chocolate to really notice its color. I smell its sweet scent and notice the tiny hint of bitter because the chocolate is so dark. I take a tiny nibble, and truly notice the taste. I pay attention to how it melts on my tongue, and how much I want another bite, a big one this time, but how savoring it makes it even better.

I eat my square, small bite by small bite, and make it last. The flavor takes over my mouth for more than just a moment like usual when I gobble the square whole. I am truly in this moment. The chocolate isn't an afterthought when my full attention is placed on it. It is my only thought.

Doing this allows me to take a mini mental vacation from the world, where I am truly immersed in my activity at hand—enjoying my chocolate. How many times do we eat something, even something we have craved and looked forward to, hardly tasting it or appreciating it?

My answer to that question is, all the time. Mindful eating falls into the category for me of "teach what you need to learn!" I know all the tools, I teach others, but I practice sporadically.

It is easier for me to eat mindfully when I am alone. I do a quick body scan to be sure I am not holding tension in my body because I know that makes me eat faster. I take a moment to bless my food, and I put my fork down between bites. Somehow this all falls apart when I am eating with other people!

I don't beat myself up about it, I simply aim to do better. The more I eat mindfully when I am alone, the more I will solidify these habits so I can continue around others. It's a process for sure, and it won't be an overnight one for me!

Lots of foods are great to use in a mindful eating exercise. Fruits and vegetables are especially good. The juice and the crunch give you a lot to focus on, and you are getting your vitamins as an added bonus to your mental health and focus.

If you want to try your own mindful eating exercise, here are the steps:

1. Get your food ready, just a small piece, not an entire meal for this exercise (that comes later!). Place it in front of you on the table.

2. Sit down in a quiet place.

3. Close your eyes.

4. Take a few nice, long, deep breaths.

5. Open your eyes and look at your food. Really notice the colors.

6. Pick up your food and notice the texture. Touch it to your lips and feel the texture.

7. Take a small nibble. Hold it in your mouth and really taste it. Name the adjectives you think of, at least three to five. Keep it in your mouth as long as possible.

8. Take another bite and notice the flavors and textures in your mouth. Chew slowly.

9. Continue eating slowly and taking a deep breath between bites. Put the food down between bites so you can truly savor, instead of rushing to put the next bite in.

10. When you are finished, take three more nice, long, deep breaths.

See how this exercise differs for you if you are eating berries, a cucumber, or chocolate.

Meditation #25

Candle Meditation

Two ways to use this

If I asked you to visualize a relaxing scene in your mind, it would most likely involve things like a bubble bath, a good book and a couch, and probably a candle.

We can use a candle in two ways to help us relax. The first is to actually light one. You can spend one minute focusing on the dance of the flame and the scent, if the candle has one. This intense concentration will calm the mind, lessen internal chatter, and bring you back to center.

Now, what if you aren't at home or somewhere appropriate to light a candle? You still can in your mind!

Visualization is a powerful tool. As long as you are in a safe, comfortable place (never driving!), close your eyes and imagine a candle in your mind's eye. Really get a sense of it. Just like with a real candle, see the flicker of the flame. See the dance of shadows on a wall. If your favorite candle has a scent, see if you can almost smell it.

This visualization tool will keep you completely in the present moment for a minute, so that when you open your eyes you will feel more centered and grounded.

Meditation #26

Be the Observer

Hmmmm . . . that's interesting

The more I become the observer of my thoughts, the more I see and notice, and the more I learn about myself every day. I don't just notice how I feel, but I investigate *why*. I feel comfortable asking myself hard questions, and understanding that I may not like everything I find out, but I am ready to know what wounds still need to heal and where I have room to grow.

It's easier to go through life without this knowledge, to coast and ignore, but that no longer feels comfortable to me. I want to work on the hard stuff! I know on the other side of "sometimes uncomfortable" is more peace, love, and acceptance. I want as much of that as I can get.

I have started saying the same thing in my head when I notice reactions of judgment, annoyance, or resentment toward another person. Instead of berating myself for having the thought or emotion because it isn't mindful or nice, I say, "Hmmm . . . that's interesting." It's interesting that I am reacting this way. Where is it coming from? What do I need to work on around this?

Here's a perfect example:

I was recently in a training class and we shared thoughts on a topic in a small group setting. I was proud of what I shared and my group members felt that it really resonated with them. I love sharing and was happy to make a valuable contribution to our group.

At the end of sharing we reconvened in our large group as a class to discuss. Someone from my small group shared my thoughts as her own to the group. My first reaction inside was "Are you freaking kidding me?!" I was a little bit in shock, and I was kind of annoyed and pissed. But those feelings felt terrible to me. So I said to myself, *Hmmm, that's interesting that I feel this way. Why, and where is it coming from?*

In all honesty it wasn't that big of a deal. I don't think this person was malicious at all, and what I said resonated with her and she wanted to share it. Of course she could have given me credit, but was that really the important part?

Once I observed and investigated my feelings I could see a bit more clearly that I do like getting credit. I like to be recognized for what I do and say. In this case though, what felt more important than getting credit was that I truly had an impact on this woman's life. What I said mattered to her, and shed new light on her thinking. That's why I love to teach and share. Is it always about credit? Why is the credit so important to me? Do I need it to fill me up? These are the types of questions I ask myself, like a reporter.

People "borrow" from me all the time. This is part of being in the public eye, and I have to investigate my feelings around it quite often. It is always nice to be quoted or given credit for an idea, and when it happens I am grateful. When it doesn't, I have a choice to make. Do I want it to drive me insane and completely ruin my day, or do I want to graciously acknowledge what an impact I am having on the world? I choose option two because it feels so much better, and it is a more heart-centered way to live. As humans, we are constantly battling ego thoughts, and trust me, I am as human as everyone else when it comes to this, but investigating these feelings and sorting through them helps me to move through them so much faster. I could have stayed pissed at that woman for days, but then I just would have lost days of peace. Is that worth it?

Next time you have uncomfortable thoughts or feelings, act like an investigator. Ask yourself hard questions, dig, and find and face wounds that, once healed, will give you so much more peace in your life. It isn't always easy, but it is always worth it.

Meditation #27

Slow Breath

Take it sloooow

There are a few earth angels that I have been blessed to work with over the years. You know about Traci (see page 109), and now I will tell you about Amy Mercree. Amy is a psychic medium and a medical intuitive. I was first introduced to her by my dear friend Kate Snowise via her podcast *Here to Thrive*. I was a guest of Kate's when *Hot Mess to Mindful Mom* first came out and we totally clicked and now I treasure our friendship.

I listened to the episode that Kate did with Amy and immediately felt connected to her relatability and authenticity. I booked an appointment with her because something told me that I needed to talk to her.

There are no coincidences, only synchronicities, and as these things usually go, my dog Hunter, who blessed our home for almost sixteen years, and I considered my firstborn, passed away just a few days before my call with Amy. Amy was able to connect me to Hunter's soul and let me know that he had transitioned with ease. I had booked the appointment weeks before we even knew Hunter was sick, but the timing was so perfect. I was devastated and this brought me so much peace.

I had a feeling that my own intuitive gifts were beginning to open. One night I had a dream that I opened my coat closet downstairs and there was a dazzling trench coat made of diamonds and sequins that sparkled more than anything I'd ever seen. I heard a voice in my head that said, "This is what you are to put on when you communicate with spirit." Talk about a sign! And there were many more.

I wanted to do whatever I could to help my gifts open as much as possible. I was on the hunt for a mentor to help me through this process, and Amy popped into my head. I knew she was the right person to help me, and we began having bi-monthly sessions together. Amy has taught me many Shamanic techniques and has led me to have unbelievable journeys into alternate dimensions. It has been a cool and crazy journey!

Before one of my journeys Amy guided me to take Straw Breaths, and I loved the practice and began teaching my clients. I have one teen client that especially loved it! It's easy and can be done anywhere.

How to take straw breaths:
1. Sit comfortably with your eyes open or closed.
2. Take a big, comfortable breath in through your nose and feel your belly rise.
3. Exhale through your mouth as slowly as possible like you are pushing air out through a straw.
4. Repeat three to five times.

This is an extremely calming breath that adults and kids all love. Try this one at a traffic light instead of reaching for your phone!

Meditation #28

Protective Light

Directly from an earth angel

The last earth angel I am going to introduce you to is Lisa Devine. Lisa has been a breath of fresh air into my last year. Believe it or not, I also heard her on Kate's podcast and fell in love with her story and spirit. (Hint, hint: download the podcast *Here to Thrive*. You won't be sorry!)

Lisa is an intuitive, focusing on connection to the archangels. I have had so many personal revelations and so much spiritual growth this year, as well as exciting business developments, and it has been comforting and helpful to have Lisa to bounce ideas off of—and of course input from the angels never hurts!

Lisa taught me a super fast way to protect my energy, and since I like options and variety, I like using this mixed in with other techniques such as using my pendulum and clear intention.

We did this quick and simple practice on the end of one or our calls, and it has always stuck with me. It is protecting our energy with a bubble of light, and even though I have done many variations of this exercise, this was the fastest and easiest, making it a perfect one-minute meditation.

How to protect with a light bubble:

1. Close your eyes and take a few nice, long, deep breaths through your nose.
2. Inhale through your nose and imagine a tiny ball of light in your heart.
3. On your next exhale, blow all the air out of your mouth, and imagine the light getting bigger and filling up your body.
4. Inhale again, and on your next exhale, as you blow the air out of your mouth, imagine this beautiful light expanding and surrounding your body and protecting your energy.
5. Set the intention that this light will protect you from any negativity throughout your day.

You can boost your light bubble as you need to during the day. Before you enter any situation, whether it be a meeting, a phone call, or a class or playdate for your kids, take one moment to breathe, and see that bubble of protective light around you. You can always blow it up again if you need to.

Kundalini Yoga Techniques
How I get sparkly and shiny

I was first introduced to Kundalini Yoga as taught by Yogi Bhajan*
by Gabby Bernstein years ago. In her videos, classes, and live events
she shared a few of the more simple meditations and techniques and
I immediately fell in love with the practice.

Of course I wanted to learn more and do more. I joke about this
with a former client of mine when we occasionally catch up. We are
both addicted to learning. I have actually had a few clients become
interested in teaching mindfulness meditation, which makes me feel
so good because I know that our work together has impacted them
in such profound ways that now they want to share it with others
too.

I began doing Kundalini classes by video from a famous studio
in New York City and Los Angeles, and then I finally found a studio
in Houston, and I began attending weekly classes there.

I felt such a difference in my energy levels, overall outlook, and
aura when I practiced Kundalini consistently in addition to my daily
seated mindfulness meditation practice. I joked that it made me feel
shiny and sparkly. People occasionally started telling me that I had a
glow. I came to value my practice so much that when a teacher training was announced at my studio in Houston it was an immediate
"hell yes!" from me. I knew that Kundalini Yoga was the next step
for me as a teacher.

When I told Mark that I wanted to get trained in Kundalini he
immediately asked me if that had something to do with sex. He was

clueless, but as always incredibly supportive, and encouraged me to go for it.

The training required two hundred hours away from my family over eight months. The timing was terrible! Adam's Bar Mitzvah was in the second month, I had to meet Mark and the boys a day late on a family vacation, and I had to miss a training weekend for a dear friend's son's Bar Mitzvah. We were only allowed to miss one weekend, and if we missed more we couldn't graduate. So before I even started training my weekend was accounted for, which meant no getting sick and no emergencies. I just willed the Universe to cooperate! Not to mention, there would be a ton of makeup work to do for the weekend I missed. Even with all this, I knew I had to move forward.

This also meant I was going to miss a few of the boys' games and activities, which is always hard, and Mark was going to have to do double duty on my training weekends. Emotionally, it was trying at times. It makes me really sad to miss anything for my kids, but I had to really think about what they would remember long-term. Would that game I missed stick out in their memory, or the fact that I went after my dreams and served the world? I banked on the latter!

I became passionate about teaching Kundalini Yoga because just like meditation it had a huge impact on my life and the way I feel day to day. My intention as a teacher is to do exactly what I did with mindfulness meditation. I want to make the concepts of Kundalini Yoga feel accessible and relatable to many people, so they learn and think, *I can do that!*

So, what is Kundalini Yoga?

Kundalini means awareness. Kundalini Yoga is the technology to awaken that awareness so that you can live your full potential. The

process of personal growth and development through Kundalini Yoga helps you unfold into your true nature, releasing whatever fear and blocks are holding you back. This practice helps you become more of who you really are, gaining new perspectives and habits to support your expanded awareness and growth.

I find that the combination of movement, mantra, meditation, and breathwork done when practicing Kundalini is so effective at creating change in my body, mind, and spirit.

I practice Kundalini Yoga as taught by Yogi Bhajan° because it helps me learn to ride the waves of life and embrace change. It also has helped my body become stronger because it boosts the immune system, glandular function, and circulation. It helps you live a more heart-centered life and release doubt and insecurity.

As Yogi Bhajan, who brought Kundalini to the West, puts it, "What is Kundalini actually? It is your creative potential. You experience it when the energy of the glandular system combines with the energy of the nervous system to create such a sensitivity that the totality of the brain receives signals and integrates them. Then you become totally and wholly aware, and your creative potential becomes available to you."

A Kundalini Yoga class as taught by Yogi Bhajan° is made up of Kriyas, or sets of exercises, meditations, pranayams (breathwork), and relaxation. I am going to share a few wonderful breathwork exercises with you that can easily be done as a beginner, and in short periods of time.

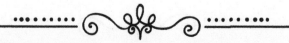

Meditation #29

Alternate Nostril Breathing

Alternate nostril breathing has many benefits, such as:
- Balancing the left and right hemispheres of the brain
- Creating a deep sense of well-being and harmony on the physical, mental, and emotional levels
- Helping with headaches, migraines, and other stress-related issues

How to do it:
1. Keep your breath deep and relaxed.
2. Sit in a chair with your feet on the floor or on the floor in easy pose (cross-legged).
3. Have your left hand resting on your left thigh if you are in a chair, or on your left knee if you are in easy pose, with your thumb and forefinger touching. This is called Gyan Mudra. (A mudra is a position of the hands that seals and guides energy flow and reflexes the brain.)
4. You will be alternating which nostril you breathe out of— Use the thumb of the right hand to close the right nostril and when time to switch, the index finger or ring finger of the

right hand to close the left nostril. Before you begin, practice switching which nostril you close for just a moment. When you are comfortable with the movement, move to step #5.

5. Close the right nostril and gently and fully inhale through the left nostril.
6. Then close the left nostril and exhale through the right nostril.
7. Then inhale through the right nostril.
8. Close the right nostril and exhale through the left nostril.
9. Continue repeating, alternating nostrils after each inhalation.

I once took a class where we did an advanced move. You can try it if you are ever up for a challenge! After you do alternate nostril breathing for a minute, you can drop your hands and see if you can keep the breath pattern going just by feel. It's definitely hard!

Meditation #30

Single Nostril Breathing

It's also extremely helpful that you can use single nostril breathing in a more prescriptive manner like this.

If you need to relax: Use your right thumb to cover your right nostril and just breathe in and out of your left nostril for a minute.

This helps us become more calm in the moment, more sensitive, and more empathetic. This is a great way to calm down in any stressful situation, and even before bed.

If you need more energy: Use your left thumb to cover your left nostril and just breathe in and out of your right nostril for a minute.

This is an invigorating breath that can help you to feel more alert, and help us concentrate. Use this before working on a project, or when you feel your energy slump in the afternoon.

Meditation #31

Four-Stroke Breath

With segmented breaths we divide the inhale and exhale into several equal parts. In this exercise we will divide each into four equal parts which can aid us in feeling more clarity and alertness and can help trigger the glandular system.

There is a slight suspension of the breath between each part and a distinct beginning and end point to each segment. Instead of inhaling in one smooth motion, we break the breath into segmented "sniffs." Try not to collapse or squeeze the nostrils on the inhalation or pull the breath too deeply into the lungs. The goal is for the breath to strike a more relaxed, yet focused area in the nasal passage, in turn stimulating particular nerves. Keep the nostrils relaxed and direct your attention to the feel of the breath further along the air passages and to the motion of the diaphragm.

When you breathe, separate each inhale and exhale into four separate and equal parts. One inhalation and exhalation equals four short yet distinct sniffs. Four in, four out.

If you want to try other ratios, please consult a Kundalini Yoga teacher. Not all ratios are balanced or sustainable, so don't guess!

If you want to find out more about Kundalini Yoga as taught by Yogi Bhajan®, or find a teacher and classes in your area, please visit www.3ho.org or www.kundaliniresearchinstitute.org.

Great one-minute meditations for kids

Kids are more stressed than ever these days, so they need and want one-minute meditations as much as we adults do! With kids, especially little ones, I like to keep it light and fun. I personally start working with kids in my private practice at ten years old, but lots of my clients have small children and want ideas for how to introduce the concepts of meditation into their lives. These are the tools that I have shared with great success. I get rave reviews on them.

Meditation #32

Balloon in the Belly

I instruct my clients during parts of meditation to really breathe into their belly, or to take "belly breaths." The easiest way to understand how to do this is to imagine you are blowing up a balloon in your belly in the inhale, and then let all the air out of the balloon on the exhale.

Kids usually love balloons so this is a great visualization for them. They can pick their favorite color to make it even more fun and give them some autonomy in the exercise. They can simply imagine blowing up and releasing the balloon for a minute, or as long as they want.

You can also guide them to take this practice one step farther in two different ways.

Let go of a worry

If they have something weighing on their mind, or are feeling anxious, overwhelmed, frustrated, or stressed in any way, on the last inhale of the practice they can imagine putting their worry inside of the balloon. On the exhale they can imagine their balloon floating into the blue sky with their worry inside, carrying it far, far away. This is a great release.

Make a wish

They can also imagine a wish filling the balloon on their last inhale, and on their last exhale the balloon can carry their wish up into the sky. You can take this as far as you or your kids like, by saying their wish will go to God, or the angels, or you can use whatever words would bring them comfort. Every household has different preferences for this.

Belly breathing is a wonderful way to help kids relax during the day, or before bed. Use this tool with your kids, and after a few practice sessions with you, they will be able to do it on their own whenever they need to.

Meditation #33

Good Night with a Crystal

Using a body scan before bed can be a great way to help your kids release any residual tension that may be lingering in their body so that they can fall asleep faster and with a calmer nervous system.

My boys love to be guided through a body scan before bed. Refer to page 77 for a meditation to help your kids complete a body scan.

A dear friend told me that her daughter was having a lot of trouble falling asleep. I wanted to think of something really special that she could do with her to help. It can be hard to think on the spot, but I had a precious download with an inpired idea that her daughter really loved. Since then I have shared this tool with others and kids really seem to take to it. This is a body scan with a little twist!

I suggested that my friend get a beautiful crystal in a color that her daughter would love. You can find them at metaphysical bookstores, or even online. Your child can also pick one out themselves if you think it would make the process more exciting for them.

This crystal is the "Magic Sleep Crystal" and it helps them say good night to each part of their body before bed. I instructed my friend to have her daughter get comfy in bed, ready to go to sleep.

She then put the magic sleep crystal on each main part of her daughter's body to "say good night." I suggested that she include all the parts of the face, the neck, shoulders, arms, hand, chest, belly, legs, and feet. You can be as simple or as detailed as you want. You can say "foot" or do each individual toe. Up to you. Every time the crystal touched a body part they said, "Good night, _____."

This is a fun and lighthearted way to make a meditation technique really accessible and enjoyable for kids. I would not be surprised if some nights you never even made it to the feet before they are asleep!

Meditation #34

Lovie on the Belly

This is another variation on belly breathing that is fun for kids and feels like a game.

If your child has something special that is small enough to lay on their belly, I suggest using that. If they don't have a blanket or stuffed animal that's special to them, choose a small toy or animal that can fit on their belly.

Have them lie down on their bed, the couch, or the floor, and place their lovie or special animal on their belly. Encourage them to watch their lovie move up and down as they breathe and see how many rides they can give before the lovie falls off.

I had one rambunctious boy do this exercise with action figures. Whatever works! They won't even realize that they are taking deep breaths but they will feel so much better after. You can put one on your belly and do it with them, too. Really make it feel like a fun game. You can even set it up like a challenge—who in the family can keep their stuffed animal on the longest?

If you want to use belly breathing with your child when you are out and about or in the car and you don't have props, but you want variation from the balloon, you can also encourage them to place their hand on their belly, right under their belly button, and see if they can watch their hand move up and down ten times.

Meditation #35

Matching Inhale and Exhale

I teach matching your inhale and exhale to everyone I see in my practice, teach online, or pretty much just come into contact with, because it is so doable. I get asked all the time at cocktail parties and luncheons, and even in line at the grocery store, how to meditate. There is so much to say on the topic, but when I need to give a one-minute quick tip, I use "matching the inhale and exhale."

The basic is just to inhale and silently count to three in your head and then match that silent count of three as you exhale. Pause, and do it right now. See? Pretty simple!

Kids can catch on to this breath pattern very easily and take to it usually the very first time. They can do it as a teacher is passing out a test or if they feel anxious or overwhelmed. It is just as easy to do with eyes open or closed.

There are also ways to spruce it up for kids who are visual learners so that it feels more fun. Try teaching your kids this technique: *Imagine sitting on a beautiful beach and watching a wave rolling into the shore as you inhale and count to three, and then rolling back out to sea as you exhale and count to three.*

If they are really into dinosaurs or the solar system, or the

circus, or ballet, get creative and incorporate what they like into the exercise.

I talk a lot more about introducing your kids to meditation in my second book, *Get the Most out of Motherhood*. Definitely get a copy if you want more on this topic!

SECTION 3

Moving Forward with Ease and Grace

Now that you are armed with all these new tools, it can feel a little overwhelming. You may be asking, "What now?" The key is to move forward with ease and grace. Don't put too much pressure on yourself. Give yourself permission to integrate these tools slowly into your life. It is obviously impossible to use thirty-five new tools at once, so pick one, two, or three that you gravitate toward and start with those. As you feel ready to incorporate more into your life, do so. There is no timeline for success. You have there rest of your life to use them!

In the following chapters you will discover ways to bring these tools to your family, more ways to empower yourself in terms of change, and additional tips for how and when to practice. I have also included answers to the most frequently asked questions about meditation. It felt so good to compile them in one place!

The most important thing to remember is to be kind and compassionate toward yourself when you are learning and practicing anything new. If you make that a priority, you can't go wrong.

Chapter 8

Make It a Family Affair

Model, Model, Model!

> The Golden Rule of Parenting; do unto your children
> as you wish your parents had done unto you.
> —LOUISE HART, AUTHOR

People are constantly asking me how to get their kids to meditate. My very first question to them is, do *you* meditate? Children are great at imitating us. They are the mirror for every bad word we've ever said! So let's give them every positive example that we can.

Our kids pay much more attention to what we do than what we say. We can preach to them all day long but trust me, they are watching our actions and words.

If we talk to our kids about how important it is to eat healthy, and we are chomping on chips all day long, think they will listen?

If we tell our kids not to curse, but bad words are flying out of our mouths all day long, think they will listen?

If we tell our kids how important it is to take deep breaths when they are stressed, and they see us do it, think they will listen?

Yes! Maybe I got you on the last one.

I will never forget the very first time I saw my oldest take deep breaths when he felt stressed, unprompted by me. The only reason he knew to do that is because he had seen me do it, probably hundreds of times, and he caught on.

If you want your kids to grow up thinking exercise, eating well, getting enough sleep, and using one-minute meditations are important, then set a good example. You are setting the tone for your home, so take advantage of the gift you have—their attention. They *are* paying attention.

This doesn't mean that we as parents have to be perfect all the time. It isn't possible even if we tried, but our children can see us putting our best foot forward each and every day. When we do fall off our routines, getting right back on to them is a lesson for our kids too. It's not about beating ourselves up for what we didn't do, it's about moving forward in the most nourishing way possible.

In order for our kids to learn from us, we have to talk about our practices with them. Let them know you meditate and use one-minute meditations when you feel stressed. Let them know at a traffic light that you are making a conscious choice to not pick up your phone, but to breathe instead. When you feel overwhelmed, frustrated, sad, or stressed, let them occasionally know, and tell them what tool you are using to come back to center. We want our kids to have these tools, but we can't expect them to magically develop them without an example and guidance.

We are also showing our kids that we have a range of emotions just like they do. In fact, all humans do, and even though some of the feelings we have aren't the most fun, they are normal. We can't control every situation in life, but we can control how we respond to it.

I have some clients that have instituted a short family meditation time each night. I have one client that climbs into bed each night and meditates with her daughter. I have other clients who lead their young kids by example, creating an environment in their home where meditation is normal and just something that people do. Their young kids won't remember a different way.

No matter what feels right to you, any exposure to self-care and self-help tools is a huge gift that you can give your children. Talk about the ways you take care of yourself in normal, everyday conversation. Make it a part of your family vocabulary. Even if your kids don't immediately pick up the tools, you are embedding them into their knowledge base to use anytime that feels right for them.

Chapter 9

Empower Yourself to Never Feel Stuck

There Is Always a Tool

> I realized that I don't have to be perfect. All I have to do is show up and enjoy the messy, imperfect, and beautiful journey of my life.
> —KERRY WASHINGTON, ACTRESS

When I look at the growth that I have sustained over the past seven years of prioritizing my health—body, mind, and spirit—I am overcome with pride and self-love. I know I am a better mom, wife, friend, sister, daughter, teacher, coach, and an all-around better *me*. I am more compassionate, less reactive, and I have a better handle on my anxiety. I lead by example, and feel one of my greatest gifts in this lifetime is the honor of inspiring others to live a better life. There is one specific area of my life, however, that mindfulness hasn't infiltrated. My spending.

Some background: I am a total girlie girl. I love makeup, clothes,

face products, and hair products. I love trying new things and sharing my latest obsessions with my friends and family. When I love something, I want to tell everyone about it. If I didn't go the mindfulness route in my career, I could have been a beauty blogger!

I have mastered the mindful pause when it comes to reacting to situations that make me feel uncomfortable or responding to texts and emails. I have learned to breathe through my fears and not be scared of putting myself out there. I can get up in front of a crowd, give a speech, and leave the audience feeling inspired and excited. But I can't say "no" when I am shopping. There is no pause before I click "buy" or swipe my card.

I have never gone into debt, or spent more than I could afford, but I have had lots of cases of buyer's remorse and looked at barely-worn clothes in my closet that I should have left at the store. These moments make me feel wasteful and frustrated, and I want to move forward purchasing things when I have put actual thought into it instead of mindlessly buying.

I was determined to bring more mindfulness into my consumption, and in order to make this a reality, I did a six-month experiment of no spending on clothes or products. Here's how I came up with the idea.

I had been drawn to reading books like *Soulful Simplicity* by Courtney Carver, and *The Year of Less* by Cait Flanders. These are memoirs of people who have decluttered their lives and decided to live with less. When I looked at the supplements under my bathroom sink that I don't use, and the various things in my kitchen cabinets that haven't seen the light of day in ten years, I wanted them out. Clothes that I don't ever wear are starting to depress me, and life is definitely too short for that! I wanted to declutter my life!

I felt like I need more room to breathe. I wanted to tackle

decluttering my home, as well as becoming a more mindful consumer. I needed to practice saying "no" and simply being more grateful for the abundance that I already had in my life. I wanted less time in stores and more time in nature. I wanted less time thinking about buying things and more time hugging my kids. That was why I came up with doing my own mindful spending experiment.

The authors of the books I read usually did their experiments for a year, but that felt overwhelming so I started with six months and decided to take it from there. I was originally going to do three, but it didn't feel like enough time to really solidify my new habits.

I decided I needed some guidelines for myself so I came up with a few ground rules:

1. No purchasing clothing, shoes, or purses.
2. I could replenish self-care items like cosmetics or lotions if the bottle or tube runs out, but I couldn't buy anything new to try.
3. I couldn't purchase random crap on Amazon because it's easy and one-click buying feels like fake money.
4. I could buy whatever the kids need or we legitimately need for our home. This was about me and *my* habits!
5. No new self-help books during this experiment because I had a stack that I hadn't read yet, but I could buy fiction. This was great timing anyway as it gave me time to finish this book, and I never read self-help while I am writing my own self-help book!
6. I could still get mani/pedis, but my place is ridiculously expensive, so I switched to one that costs less and felt a bit more reasonable.
7. I pre-approved a few items to purchase that I had been on the lookout for. I had permission to buy two bathing suits

and one new cover-up for summer, as well as one white long sleeve. That's it.

8. I could purchase gifts for others.
9. My birthday was in the middle of the experiment. My husband could buy me a gift but I couldn't ask for anything specific.

I decided to keep a running list of products, clothes, and books that I wanted to evaluate at the end of experiment. I called it the "Want List!" I thought it would be interesting to see what I still care about purchasing a few months later. I am assuming (and hoping) not much! I told myself that if there was really something that I still wanted from the Want List at the end of the experiment, I could have it then.

I knew going into the experiment that the grocery store was a place I'd have to be careful, especially Whole Foods. Products there are still products!

The crazy thing is that when I told people in my newsletter and on social media that I was doing the Mindful Spending Experiment, I got tons of feedback from people who wanted to do it with me. I was blown away by the response! I had at least one hundred people joining in, in their own form of the experiment. Some people did it for a shorter amount of time, and others chose a different area of their life that was a trigger for them.

I learned so much about my habits and triggers during those six months. I wasn't perfect, but I did *so* much better than I thought I would. I am so proud. Here are a few highlights of what happened and what I learned:

- In the beginning, probably for the first three weeks, I still pulled into the driveway craning my neck to simultaneously

look at the front door to see if any packages arrived. After
that, I forgot to look.

- At the beginning of the experiment a few boxes were still being
delivered for things I had ordered before it started, and when
they came I couldn't even remember what was in them. It was
eye-opening for me to understand that I ordered so much I
had no clue what anything was when the boxes arrived.

- My very favorite clothing store in the world is in the same
shopping center as Whole Foods. I am there all the time,
and for the first month I would get a little sad when I saw
the storefront because it felt forbidden. After that it stopped
bothering me; I knew in a few short months I could go if I
wanted to. This was also a chance to break my habit of pop-
ping in all the time. I know I will be more mindful about
this going forward.

- I made a note a few weeks into the experiment in my journal
about how empowered I was feeling about this journey.

- I had way less to drag to the end of my driveway for recy-
cling each week without so many boxes!

- When I wanted something I occasionally had a moment
where I first thought about hopping online to order it, but
ultimately, I always remembered to add it to the Want List.

- Each month I would reevaluate my Want List and take
things off.

- I had a crazy, crazy dream where I was shopping and I
brought all these cute dresses and rompers to the check out
and then burst into tears and started screaming, "I can't
have any of this!"

- I saw my friend wearing a shirt I loved about three weeks
in, and ordinarily I would have ordered it in about thirty

seconds flat. I had a momentary pang of want, and realized I still had work to do moving into gratitude instead of being triggered by wants.

- I bought myself a weighted blanket and blue-light glasses to help me with sleep. I was feeling really guilty and I actually evaluated this decision quite a bit, but since my arthritis flares when I am overtired, I decided that anything related to sleep was a medical expense.

- When I got my first credit card bill after the experiment started, I could already see the difference, and it felt so empowering.

- It was so fun to help other people pick out fun things—as much as getting things for myself.

- I saw my obsessive behavior surface over self-tanner. I couldn't stop thinking about it once it got really hot. I realized how ridiculous I was being about it, but it was still on my mind. I had melanoma when I was thirty-four, so I really can't sit in the sun, but I love being tanned. I decided it was a product, and it was off-limits, but then I pushed it to medical expense which, looking back, was ridiculous and I totally broke my self-imposed contract with that one . . . but I paid the price. I woke up the next morning after using it and I looked like a brown zebra with stripes all over my legs. It was totally embarrassing! I had to then have someone come to my house to spray tan me to fix it!

- Even though I wasn't supposed to, I'll fess up . . . my husband asked me for some birthday ideas and I did give him a few.

- I got so many decluttering projects done in my house as part of the experiment.

- I had a stylist help me clean out my closet, which was hugely helpful, and I began wearing clothes that I forgot about and enjoying the clothing I already owned so much more.

I enlisted a professional organizer to help me with decluttering projects, mostly to help me block off the time and commit to doing them. My house is in great shape and I feel like I can breathe better!

Those are some highlights. You can see that I wasn't perfect, but I made tons of progress. I'd say one of the biggest tools for me became the Want List, and this is something I will carry forward in my life. It may not be for six months, probably more like a week or two, but I can see how taking a mindful pause makes me really think about what I want in the moment and what I want long-term. I took almost everything off my Want List by the end of the six months because after really thinking about most things, I realized they were more fun and exciting in the moment than actually practical.

This experiment definitely made me more mindful in terms of consuming. I am truly glad I did it. It will be an ongoing process to continue to maintain my new habits, but I feel empowered by the progress that I made and so much more aware of what I still want to work on.

I shared this experiment with you to show you how creative you can be when it comes to using tools in your life. You don't have to feel stuck in a bad habit or cycle. There is always a way to empower yourself to change.

Think about what feelings you want to bring into your life, and what's holding you back from getting there. Can you do your own version of the Mindful Spending Experiment? Maybe it's something you could try for a week, or a month, or even six. It's not about becoming perfect, it's more about awareness and progress.

What do you want to change? I wanted to be more mindful with my spending, but maybe you want to change your eating habits, really bring meditation into your life, or stop yelling at your kids? How can one-minute meditations help you get there?

I used them during my experiment when I wanted to buy something and couldn't. I needed to come back to center quickly so instead of feeling deprived I could focus on gratitude.

If you want to bring more meditation into your life, set a reminder on your phone every hour to do a one-minute meditation. If you want to eat healthier, do a one-minute meditation and get a glass of water every time you crave junk food. When your kids are driving you crazy, a one-minute meditation is crucial to responding in a way that feels good to you and the kids instead of reacting in a way you will regret.

The possibilities are endless! All it takes is a bit of soul-searching to see where in your life you want to make a change. Then get creative!

Chapter 10

Trust Yourself!

Establish a Relationship with Your Soul

Learning to trust yourself means making mistakes
and loving yourself anyway.
—CHERYL RICHARDSON

We all have patterns that we follow in our lives, situations that repeatedly present themselves, and we wonder, *Why does this keep happening to me?!* Our intuition may be screaming "NOOOOO!" but we don't listen. You may be smiling to yourself right now, thinking about how you always say "yes" when you don't mean it, go for the same kind of man knowing you will get hurt, or accept jobs that don't take you further in life. Maybe you have the same fight with your teenager, even though you know what you should be doing differently yet never follow through, or allow your kids to run the show in your home even though you know what's best.

We all have our "stuff."

Even though I am blessed and grateful to have some wonderful, long-standing friendships in my life, I admittedly have a pattern of jumping into other friendships too quickly and not listening to my intuition when I am getting to know a new friend and it doesn't feel like an energetic match.

The same situation will keep coming back to haunt us unless we finally change our behavior, and I speak from experience. A few years ago, I reached the final straw with myself.

I became friends with someone even though my intuition was not only screaming "no!" but showing me red flags in my head. I felt a little off every time we got together, but I ignored the blaring warning signs and of course it didn't end well. Having a fallout with a friend is never fun, but the guilt I felt from ignoring my gut lingered long after the blowout. I'd done so much work on connecting with my higher self, but the situation made me realize I still needed to work on solidifying my new habits. I decided I owed it to myself to make this the very last time I ignored my intuition.

I thought it would be fun to do a little experiment. I decided to keep an "Intuition Journal." For one month I kept track of every signal my intuition gave me, whether it was a feeling in my gut or a thought that popped into my head. I wrote down what happened when I listened, and what happened when I didn't. This exercise completely changed my life.

Every single time that I didn't listen, I had regrets. Here are just a few examples:

- My kids were playing soccer in the living room, and I had a strong feeling I should tell them to stop, but I got distracted. One of them kicked the ball into my favorite table and broke the leg.

- Getting ready for a party, I had a feeling in my gut that I should change. I blew it off and regretted it when I entered the party and realized I was dressed inappropriately.
- I had a nudge to check my son's backpack and told myself I would do it later. My dog found his lunch, ate it, and got sick.
- I had a hunch during a workout that the weights I was using were too heavy, but I didn't listen to my body and I pulled out my back.

I quickly realized that almost all of my entries were about times that I didn't listen to my intuition, and it was an amazing visual to help me see that this needed to change. I was super smart—if I would just pay attention to myself!

Enough Is Enough!

This experiment was a turning point in my life. I gained so much awareness around my habit of second guessing myself, which led me to learn to trust myself more and understand that the signals I get from my higher self, or the Universe, or whatever you like to call it, are not random. Now whenever I get a feeling, a hunch, or an idea pops into my head, I never doubt it.

The rare occasions these days when I don't listen to my inner wisdom, and should have, are reminders that I cannot ever stop trusting the guidance that I get from my higher self and the Universe. I feel grateful every day and consider them gifts.

This process was so life-changing for me that I created a downloadable Intuition Journal for you so that you too can use this valuable tool. To get your very own, visit http://www.hotmessto mindfulmom.com/intuition-journal/

How to Use Your Own Intuition Journal

Intuition is the ability to understand something immediately, without the need for conscious reasoning. You might know it as your "gut feeling" or "instinct."

When you receive hits of information or ideas, an unexplained feeling, or a conscious knowing, this is your intuition talking to you. Some people feel that this is their highest self talking to them, and others feel that it is the Universe giving them a useful download. However you personally feel about your intuition is right for *you*.

Think of your intuition as an internal GPS system that is there to help you stay on track in every situation. Those feelings you get in your gut, or the thoughts that pop into your head, are your body's way of interpreting the information from your higher self, which if it were a GPS would say, "You are about to make a wrong turn! Stay on track!"

As human beings we have free will when it comes to listening and following through on the intuitive hits we get. Once I used this Intuition Journal for thirty days it became clear to me that these signals should not be ignored no matter how insignificant they seemed in the moment. I was receiving these hits for a reason in every situation.

Keeping track of when I listened and when I didn't was life changing for me. It made me much more aware of and in tune with my intuition, which in turn made me more confident. I want the same for you!

Give yourself thirty days of using the Intuition Journal as a gift to yourself. You have nothing to lose and so much to gain!

Using the Intuition Journal is very simple. Take note at least one time a day of when you feel your intuition kick in. You may get a feeling in your gut, or an idea may pop into your head. Bring

awareness to how your intuition speaks to *you*. This is a very individual thing, and it can happen in multiple ways in different situations. It is important to start to pay attention to any intuitive hit you get, big or small.

There is room each day in the journal to take note of what intuitive hit you got that day. Record what it was, whether you listened to it, and what happened. (If you want to record multiple experiences per day, make extra copies of the journal pages.)

It won't take long to notice patterns develop, and to quickly understand if you typically follow the intuitive guidance you receive or not. In no time you will feel much more connected to your sense of inner knowing, and more trusting of the guidance you receive. This can lead to fewer regrets in life and more confidence in your decision-making skills. You will learn to *trust yourself* in a whole new way!

This is applicable to so many different situations, but especially if you are wondering which one-minute meditation to use in the moment of stress. Listen to your intuition.

So many of us second-guess ourselves to death. You could waste so much time and energy deciding which one-minute meditation to use that you stress yourself out more!

When you know that you need to come back to center, ask yourself which tool you need in the moment, and the very first one you think of is the one you need to use. No second guessing!

You may find that you constantly gravitate toward one particular meditation, and that's totally fine. One may seem like your BFF for a period of time and then you are ready to move on. That's okay, too. You can't go wrong rotating them or sticking with one, as long as you follow your gut instinct when you choose. Learning to listen to your intuition is about trust.

Chapter 11

Practice When Calm

Practice Makes Progress

Knowledge is of no value unless you put it into practice.
—ANTON CHEKHOV

You can't use all of these tools at once! To get started, you will need to decide what practices and meditations from this book you gravitate to the most. Pick two or three and begin practicing. You can slowly keep trying more until you find your favorites. Of course you can use them all, but you want to practice your favorites to mastery. You want to have enough experience with some of the meditations that they feel easy for you to practice when you feel stressed. You want to be comfortable enough with them that you don't have to reference a book in the moment of stress. You just pull a tool out of your back pocket!

In order to gain mastery, you want to practice one-minute meditations when you are feeling calm so that they come naturally to you

in stressful situations. There is no wrong time to use them. How about:

- When you wake up
- Before bed
- In the shower
- At a traffic light
- Standing in line at the grocery store
- Standing in line at the juice bar
- In a carpool line
- Any line!
- While cooking
- Before (or after) a journaling session
- Before a meeting at work
- As you pick up your book to read
- Before you eat
- As you fold laundry
- As you walk outside

The more you use these tools and meditations when you are calm, the more effective they are when you are stressed. This is a great point to reiterate with your kids as well. You can't count on any tool to get you out of a tough spot if you've never practiced it before!

When you are practicing these tools, remember: it isn't about perfection, it's about progress and doing *your* personal best.

Compassion for yourself is key. Never underestimate its importance. If you are stressed and you forget to use a meditation, let it go! You will have plenty more chances. Beating yourself up about forgetting is the opposite of helpful.

One of my favorite zen proverbs says, "Let go or be dragged."

You have to let go of the past or it will drag you down. This 100 percent applies. Growth comes with recommitment. If you forget to use a tool in the moment of stress, simply commit to using it next time. And maybe spend a day or two doing a few extra quick meditations when you are calm just to get in a little extra practice. They will also be at the forefront of your mind the more you do them. This will help you get back into your routine of using them when you are stressed.

Please don't make it more complicated than you need to. The basics are:

- Practice your one-minute meditations when you feel calm and are going about your day.
- Let them serve you in moments of stress.

That's truly all there is to it!

Chapter 12

Ready for More?

These Can Be Just the Beginning

> The secret of change is to focus all of your energy
> not on fighting the old, but on building the new.
>
> —SOCRATES

I am so proud of you! One-minute meditations are now part of your life, and there is no turning back. Honestly, soon you won't be able to remember your life without them. The more you use them, the less anxious, frustrated, and overwhelmed you will feel, and the more centered, present, and connected you will feel. Everyday life begins to feel more manageable, more joyful, and more engaging. It might take some time to make them a habit, but little by little you'll start to feel yourself moving through stressful situations with ease. As you build up your habits, though, don't forget to be compassionate with yourself on days you fall short of your meditation goals.

I am all about meeting people where they are.

I can preach from every mountaintop and tall building about how much I love meditation and what the benefits are, and still many, many people will not feel ready to have a daily seated practice of five, ten, or twenty minutes.

What I have found through all my teaching and coaching, working with moms, and working in the corporate world, is that everyone *does* feel like they have *one minute*. I knew I was on to something, and for this reason I made one-minute meditations a cornerstone of my teaching. I was able to connect with everyone I came into contact with, whether they were the CEO of a company or CEO of their home, and get them excited about feeling less stress in their lives in a way that felt doable for them.

One-minute meditations are something you can do forever. You can teach your children, loved ones, friends, and coworkers. You can teach the person that looks stressed standing in front of you in the grocery store or your hairdresser. Spread the love! Practicing and using these meditations is a gift you are giving to yourself day in and day out.

My hope is that these quick meditations soon feel like an extension of all of your activities and become part of the natural flow as you move through your days. You may use them forever, feel great, and stay there, or maybe, just maybe, you will become curious and want to know what two minutes of meditation feels like. Then three. In time you may want a daily seated practice, and I don't want to leave you hanging with what the next step would be if that's the case.

You can do any of these one-minute meditations for longer periods of time. It's pretty simple, but you may have additional questions. I want to get ahead of some of them in order for you to feel comfortable and confident meditating for longer periods of time.

These are some of the most frequently asked questions I get when it comes to meditation:

Q: If I can't clear my mind, am I doing it wrong?
A: If I could delete one sentence from ever being spoken on earth again, it would be "Just clear your mind." This concept is virtually unattainable for most everyone, including me! When new meditators think they are supposed to clear their minds of all thought, or they are meditating incorrectly, it sets them up to fail and be disappointed, ultimately giving up on the practice.

The average human being has a thought about every two seconds, which can be the equivalent of 50,000 to 60,000 thoughts in one day. To think that you will sit down for even one or two minutes and not have any thoughts isn't realistic.

In meditation we don't have to worry about clearing our minds. Instead, our intention is to constantly refocus our attention away from stories like your grocery list or work, and stay present. We do this by using a focus, such as our breath, our body, or a mantra. There are many to choose from, and after practicing all the one-minute meditations offered here, you will have lots of options to pick from.

A focus acts as our home base. It's where we want to be during our meditation. Whenever our mind wanders, we return to our focus. No matter how many times you have to refocus your attention, meditation is working. Your only job is to notice a thought and choose to come back to your focus. Over and over.

This constant practice with refocusing our attention during our meditation practice allows us to live a better life outside of meditation. We are able to focus on what really matters to us in the moment such as our relationships, our work, or even enjoying downtime.

Take any pressure you feel about "clearing your mind" off of your shoulders, and enjoy your practice. This is a tool that will work if you work it!

Q: What time of day should I meditate?
A: When it comes to having a daily seated practice, my teacher and mentor Sarah McLean has the best line when it comes to time of day to meditate. She says, "The best time to meditate is the time you are going to do it." Simple, yet profound.

So many aspects of meditation are personal. Where you do it, how you sit, what focus you use, and also what time of day works for you.

When you are building a new habit it can help if you stay consistent with when and where you meditate. Think about your schedule. Are you an early riser? Does before bed appeal to you more? Pick one and try it. I tell all my students, "Date it before you marry it!" If you try a certain time of day and after a few days or weeks it isn't working for you, change. It's okay! When we are starting to build new habits, there is some trial and error involved.

I like to have quiet time and meditate first thing in the morning so that I begin my day from a really centered and peaceful place. I feel like then I can take that energy with me throughout my day. Other people like to hit the ground running when they wake up, so they prefer late afternoon or evening. They feel that it helps to release any tension that has built up during the day. Again, there is no right or wrong. Think about what feels good to you.

It can also feel helpful to attach meditation to another daily habit, something you already do. For me it's waking up and letting out my dogs. I do it every day! I wake up, and the first thing I do after I take my dogs out is meditate and practice Kundalini Yoga.

Other habits you could try attaching to are brushing your teeth, turning the coffee maker on, changing your clothes after work, or tucking in your kids.

Q: Does it matter where I meditate?

A: One of the best things about meditation is that it is the most portable self-help and self-care practice. You can do it anytime, anywhere! We have certainly covered this in terms of one-minute meditations, and the same concept goes for a longer practice. As long as you are safe and comfortable, you can do it anywhere. I have meditated in a bathroom stall, in a carpool line, and on the beach.

When it comes to developing a daily seated practice, which occurs mostly in your home, it can help solidify your habit if you create a sacred space for yourself. This is simply a place that you meditate in every day.

When I started meditating, my sacred space was sitting on the edge of my tub. I still can't understand why I picked that! I guess I woke up, relieved myself, and then just sat down on the closest ledge! I soon moved into my closet, which felt like a perfect little cocoon. Once I began teaching, I dedicated a room of my house to my business, so the "zen den" became my sacred space. It is my favorite room in my house!

You don't need anything special to make it sacred. It is the intention you set when you sit there that does it. So pick your favorite chair or spot on the couch and simply sit there each day.

If it makes you feel good to light a candle, place flowers, or have a favorite framed picture, then by all means do it, but those things don't add power to your meditation. They create a lovely ritual which may make sitting down to meditate even more enticing.

Some people like to use an essential oil such as lavender while they meditate, which can help you to relax into your practice a bit.

Q: What is meditation actually doing for me besides making me feel better in the moment?

A: There is so much to say here, but I will have to settle for giving you some highlights.

There are so many physical, mental, and spiritual benefits of having a consistent meditation practice. Here are a few:

Physical:
- Helps regulate sleep patterns
- Helps improve digestion
- Helps boost the immune system
- Lowers blood pressure, cholesterol, and cortisol
- Increases energy as it helps to reduce stress

Mental:
- Improves memory, creative thinking, and clarity
- Reduces reactivity, increases responsive behavior
- Increases self-compassion and confidence
- Reduces fear and anxiety
- Improves emotional control

Spiritual:
- Increases connection to your intuition
- Connects you to the world around you
- Heightens your sense of peace and balance
- Enlivens compassion and empathy
- Helps connect you to a purpose

Don't they all sound amazing? I always tell my clients that I can't guarantee what will happen for them when they meditate, but I *can* guarantee they'll like it. I've never heard anyone say, "I liked myself better before I started meditating!"

Meditation also trains your attention to focus on one thing at a time, to spend more time in the present moment instead of the past or future, and to focus inward. Our lives are so busy and full, which is wonderful for many reasons, but our self-care often gets pushed to the bottom of our list. Our meditation time becomes a gift that we give to ourselves each day. It's a few minutes of peace and calm just for you.

We only have so much attention to go around, kind of like having a certain amount of money in the bank. When we use it, it's gone. Let's spend from our attention bank in ways that truly matter to us, such as connecting with loved ones, doing meaningful work, volunteering, and nourishing ourselves with self-care.

Q: Can I meditate lying down?

A: I get asked this a lot, and it's a great question. Here's the deal: you can, but unless you have a physical reason why sitting up is uncomfortable, I recommend sitting up. We have been trained our entire lives to go to sleep when we lie down, so if we are the least bit tired (and who isn't most days?) we are likely to fall asleep as soon as we close our eyes, even if our intention is to meditate.

If I am leading an extended body scan, or a yoga nidra, I have my clients lie down, but otherwise I always encourage them to sit up.

That being said, I have a few clients that come to my group classes that really like to lie down. It's a habit they formed before learning with me, and I want them to be comfortable practicing, so they lie down. It's not a make-or-break thing. If you really want to try lying down, and you fall asleep, then sit up.

If your goal is to fall asleep because you are meditating right before bed, obviously you will be lying down—that's the one time I say it is okay!

Q: How long until I notice that I feel different?
A: There is truly no right or wrong answer to this question, because it is different for everyone. I can only share my personal experience as an example, but there is absolutely no timeline as to what should happen with consistent meditation and when.

When I began meditating seven years ago, I set my timer for eight minutes a day. To be completely honest, I was so green. I hadn't done any research, and I didn't even know there were benefits of meditation, so I had no expectations.

I remember walking my dog after I had been meditating for six weeks, and I stopped short. I realized that the ball of anxiety that lived in my chest, and had for as long as I could remember, was gone. I felt so free. The only difference in my life was that I had been meditating, so I thought maybe it was doing something and I stayed extremely consistent. Within a few more weeks and the upcoming months, I began to notice that I felt calmer, less reactive, more patient with my kids, more present, more compassionate toward myself, and a bit less judgmental of others. I felt so good during the day that I decided to use extra meditations at night and a certain journaling procedure (it's in *Hot Mess to Mindful Mom*) to get off sleeping pills. Talk about life-changing! Once I learned how to fall asleep on my own I decided meditation was the best thing that ever happened to me!

Q: Why do I need to use a timer?
A: It sounds very relaxing to just sit down and go for it when you

meditate, but I promise you will want to look at the clock every minute or more if you do. It is actually more relaxing to set a timer and then meditate until it goes off. It's like you set it and forget it!

Another reason that a timer is helpful is because you want to finish every meditation you start. This is a very important concept, and the reason is this: there will inevitably be a meditation that you don't want to finish. If you are meditating for ten minutes, around five or six you will start thinking about everything you have to do and decide you don't have time. You may even feel a little stressed. Even if this is the case, you want to come back to your breath or whatever your focus is, calm yourself, refocus your attention, and finish your meditation. In doing so you will deal with stress in a calm, safe, comfortable situation, so when you are in the real world in an uncomfortable situation you will have had more practice dealing with stress and remaining calm.

I use an app called Insight Timer to time all of my meditations. I like how easy it is to use and that it has a huge library of guided meditations if I ever want to use one. You can search Ali Katz and find me and I can guide you through a few meditations!

Q: What should I actually do while I meditate?
A: I am going to break it down into some simple steps for you!

1. Find a quiet and comfortable space.
2. Take a few deep breaths and decide what your focus will be for this session.
3. Sit in a comfortable position in a chair with your feet on the floor, or cross-legged.
4. Start your timer.

5. Close your eyes and begin to breathe in and out of your nose. (If your nose is stuffy, breathe in and out of your mouth.)

6. Take a few more nice, long, deep breaths.

7. Do a quick body scan to be sure you aren't holding tension anywhere in your body.

8. Use your focus (i.e. your breath or a mantra) until your timer goes off the first time.

9. Give yourself a short one-minute integration period where you relax and enjoy the silence while your body integrates all the good you just did in your meditation. This is also a wonderful time to practice gratitude or say your own quiet prayer.

10. When your timer rings for a final time, you are finished.

11. Celebrate you and all of the good you just did for your body, mind, and spirit!

Q: What is the difference between guided meditation and meditating on my own?

A: This is a great question, and one I get often. This will be a personal choice for you, but let me share what I tell all my clients about this.

I guide people in meditation for a living, so I am obviously a fan! My goal, however, is to empower my clients to not need me forever. I work with them so they can have a successful meditation practice on their own without me, and here's why: meditation is the most portable self-help and self-care tool there is. You can meditate anywhere at any time. If you can breathe, you can meditate, so basically if you are alive, you have what you need to practice.

I encourage all my clients to meditate on their own with a timer, and to use guided meditation occasionally as a treat, or to learn or practice with a new focus.

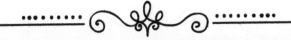

There are certain meditations like yoga nidra (yogic sleep) that must be guided. It's one of my very favorites!

That being said, if you refuse to meditate without an app or being guided, I'd still rather you meditate than not, so use them. I just hate for people to become dependent. What if you are somewhere and you don't have your phone? Will you feel like you can't meditate?

I invite you to sign up for my free five-day guided meditation challenge. Each day I will send an eight-minute guided meditation to your inbox so you get comfortable with a few different focuses. After practicing with me for five days, you will have all the confidence you need to set your timer and go for it! Sign up at http://www.hotmesstomindfulmom.com/5-day-Challenge/

Q: How long should I meditate?

A: Since I want you to finish every meditation you start, I recommend starting with a small amount of time and building as you feel ready. I started my practice with eight minutes a day, and it felt very doable. I have clients that start with anywhere from five to ten. Start with a time that feels comfortable for you. When you are ready for more, you will know. I don't give anyone a schedule to follow because I feel like you need to check in with your intuition, not a schedule, when it comes to increasing your session time. Trust your gut!

If you start at eight minutes, in a few weeks you may feel ready to go to nine or ten. Feel it out.

Don't lose sight of the fact that consistency is more important than how long you meditate for, so if you want to stay at ten minutes forever, but you do it every day, then great. Don't feel any pressure based on how others are practicing. You do *you*!

Q: Should my eyes be open or closed?

A: There are many ways to meditate, and they are all right. I find it easier to go within during my daily seated practice when my eyes are closed, and I think most people do. When I practice Kundalini Yoga, the eye gaze for each posture and meditation, called a dristi, is specified.

It isn't a requirement to close your eyes, but most people do. If you are practicing a specific type of meditation, like the candle meditation discussed earlier, then your eyes will be open.

Q: Should I meditate the same way every time?

A: So much about meditation is personal preference, and what focus you use is no exception. Some people like to use the same focus every single day, and others like more flexibility. I fall into the latter category.

I definitely have focuses that I gravitate toward, but I don't use the same one every single day. I like to take a few deep breaths and check in with my body, mind, and spirit. I ask myself, "What do you need today?" and the first focus that comes to mind is the one I use. I trust my intuition completely to guide me to the right one for me on any given day.

The best way to answer this for yourself is to play around and test out different focuses. Take a week or two and use a different one each day. Then take another week or two and use the same one. See if you feel it makes a difference or not. See what feels right for you. You will know.

Moving Forward

We are at the end of another journey together. One of my greatest joys in life is sharing my passion for meditation, mindfulness, and self-care with others. Thank you from the bottom of my heart for allowing me to share with you.

You have spent a few hours (or maybe a few weeks!) reading this book, which is an incredible first step, but the next step is beginning to use the tools. Don't wait! Start now. In fact, please do me this honor right now: *Close your eyes and take three deep breaths. Let one of these meditations come to mind. Whatever you think of, do it now for one minute.*

Congratulations! That was your first practice session. It felt great, right?

Think about the peace, calm, and presence you can bring to your life with these tools. Empower yourself to use them often, and let them serve you in times of stress. Allow them to move your life in the direction you want to go.

Please stay in touch! Drop by to let me know how it's going. You can find me on Instagram at @hotmesstomindfulmom and on

Facebook at Hot Mess to Mindful Mom with Ali Katz. If you'd like to connect with other like-minded moms, please join my Facebook group at Hot Mess to Mindful Mom Community. Visit my website to grab all of my tools and resources. Many of them are free as my gift to you. Find them all at www.hotmesstomindfulmom.com. If you want to dip your toes into the world of essential oils, please visit www.mydoterra.com/alikatz.

Good luck with your journey! This is only the beginning.

Acknowledgments

I could never have written three books in three years without the support of my family and friends. I am grateful for all of the special people in my life, and I am blessed to say that naming them all would constitute another book, but a few deserve extra special recognition.

Mark, I feel like the luckiest girl in the world to have you by my side. I thank God every day for your love, generosity, humor, support, and true partnership. Your willingness to do whatever it takes to help my dreams come true means the world to me.

Adam and Dylan, your pride in what I do, and enthusiasm for my projects, makes my heart sing. I pray that my example will help you one day to follow your heart, passion, and calling, and to never give up on your dreams.

Mom, Dad, Amy, Susan, and Steph, you are always there for me with words of encouragement and I could not ask for a better family. Love you all so much.

Jamie and Misha, what would a girl do without her besties? I am the luckiest.

Jodi, Lindsay, Kate, and Paige, you make entrepreneurship more fun than I ever thought it could be. I am so grateful that we have each other's support and friendship.

Traci, you have taught me so much over the years that has helped me to live my very best life. Grateful doesn't even cover it.

I truly love my clients and appreciate their trust in me. They were the guinea pigs for all of these exercises, and this book couldn't have been written without them!

Leah, you are an amazing editor, and I love how you just get me. Your expertise helps me to be a better writer, and it has been extremely special to be a team on three books!

Thank you to Skyhorse for believing in me a third time. I feel lucky to be a part of your book family.

Lacy and Gizmo, my four legged babies, thank you for sitting me with me as I wrote every page of this book. Your snuggles got me through.

To everyone reading this book, I write so that I can make the world a little bit better, and help anyone answering the call to bring more peace into their lives. These tools will change your life if you let them. As you read, know I wrote this book for YOU.